THE COMPLETE HERBAL GUIDE TO NATURAL HEALTH AND BEAUTY

Books by Dian Dincin Buchman

THE COMPLETE HERBAL GUIDE TO
NATURAL HEALTH AND BEAUTY
THE SHERLOCK HOLMES OF MEDICINE

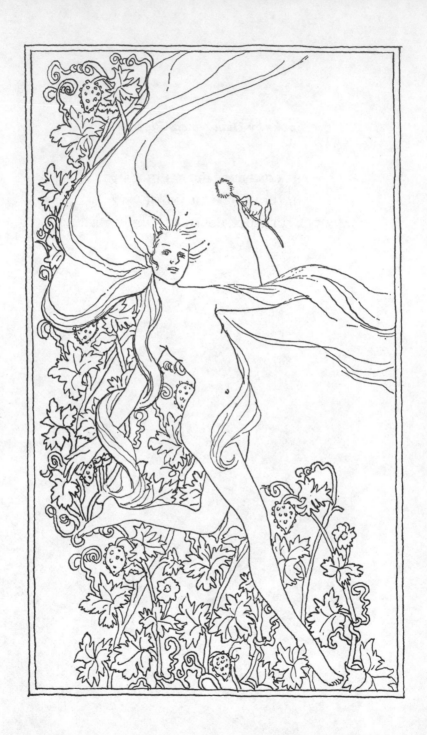

THE COMPLETE HERBAL GUIDE TO NATURAL HEALTH AND BEAUTY

DIAN DINCIN BUCHMAN

DOUBLEDAY & COMPANY, INC., GARDEN CITY, NEW YORK
1973

ISBN: 0-385-01988-2 Trade
ISBN: 0-385-08815-9 Paper
Library of Congress Catalog Card Number 73–79653

To that rare, remarkable, unusual woman,
my mother, Renee Dincin

CONTENTS

THE USEFUL PAST

I have often wondered how it is that we lost the knowledge and art of using herbs for medical and cosmetic needs. It seems strange that this lore, which was once a part of everyday life, could disappear so suddenly.

How did this change come about? A major factor was the rapid development of science in the present century, which put us in awe of anything that came out of a laboratory. We were dazzled by each new wonder drug and synthetic cosmetic, and were seduced by advertising and elegant packaging. To most of us, science seemed to herald a wonderful new world, and we rushed to scrap our grandfathers' tooth-cleaning concoctions for the delights of a tube of sweetened and flavoured paste which promised a white smile, no cavities and instant sex appeal. In a mass surrender to the need to look and be modern, we discarded indiscriminately every old-fashioned remedy, potion, simple, cream, unguent, perfume and vegetable hair dye that had been effectively used for centuries.

I remember teasing my grandmother about her collection of herbs and the time she spent preparing creams, gargles, complexion waters, pochettes and potpourris. I was embarrassed because it seemed so old-fashioned. But fortunately for me she was a nonconformist and took no notice. And I am grateful to her now for her individuality. Because I enjoyed her company, I helped her collect herbs and watched her make her creams and lotions. Thus I am able to pass on her recipes as well as the memories of herbal lore which she learned from the gypsies who lived in her remote part of Rumania.

But if we all once marched like lemmings into the modern

world, we are less innocent today. We have been alerted to the rape of our environment; we cough daily from air pollution; and we recoil in horror from hormone-injected and insecticide-ridden foods. Many of the synthetic substances we have casually used have been indicted as carcinogenic, as, for instance, with the recent furore over sodium cyclamate and products containing hexachlorophene. No doubt many other chemical mistakes will be uncovered in future.

We must therefore turn from the present and take a fresh look at the past. This can be exhilarating and fascinating, but must be done with common sense. We mustn't of course discard everything new, for that would be ridiculous. We must be selective. We must retain useful technological aids, and essential scientific data, particularly on nutrition and preventive medicine, while at the same time rediscovering what was beneficial in the past.

In writing this book, I am indebted to all the great herbalists, particularly to the English herbalists Gerard and Culpeper, the American Jethro Kloss, and the two priest-herbalists Father Kunzle of Switzerland and Father Kneipp of Germany. I have also culled the diaries of many legendary beauties of the past—Ninon de Lenclos, the Countess of Jersey, the Duchess of Alba, Lola Montez among them.

Since most people have little experience of herbs I have included a great deal of basic information. The index and chart lists each herb and pharmaceutical discussed and will demonstrate their many uses.

THE COMPLETE
HERBAL GUIDE TO
NATURAL HEALTH
AND BEAUTY

CHAPTER I

HOW TO USE HERBS

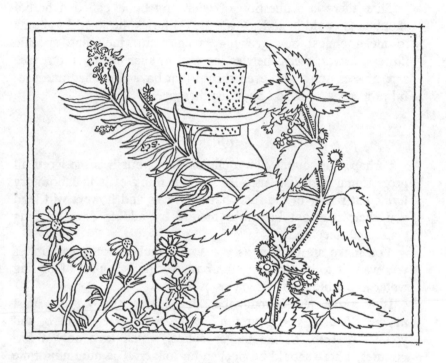

Some people can / Some people can't / Tell the difference between / Gary Cooper and Cary Grant. /

This little humorous verse somehow reminds me of the erb-herb controversy and the disparity in British and American pronunciation. For some obscure reason we Americans call herbs "erb," dropping the *h* as if we were Cockneys from the play *Pygmalion*. However we usually refer to books on this subject as herbal, and call the practitioners of the herbal craft herbalists, pronouncing the *h*'s in all these words.

I often go back and forth between the United States and Great Britain and I sometimes feel like a schizophrenic trying to adapt to each country's preferred pronunciation. I am therefore starting a one-woman movement to unite these two pronunciations into one. *H* for all of these words, please.

Then there is a question of what any book called a herbal should and could include. Over the centuries the word has come to mean almost any growing green plant, including specific flowers, leaves, seeds, berries, as well as such barks, roots, tree sap, grasses, fungi and even shrubs that have cherished and useful properties for food or botanic therapy.

Infusion

Perhaps this sounds like a clinical term, but it is the word all professional herbalists use. But do not think of it in laboratory terms but rather of the fact that all leaves and flowers will lend you their personal identities merely by adding some boiling water and steeping.

You make an infusion as you would make strong tea. Unless you want it to be stronger, the basic recipe is 1 pint of boiling water to 2 tablespoons of leaves or flowers.

It is important to remember that leaves and flowers must *never be boiled*. You pour the boiling water *over* the herb, and you let it steep. Unlike tea or coffee, which take only a few minutes, a herb should be steeped far longer. The minimum time for cosmetic use (it takes longer for medicinal use) is 15 minutes, but the longer you allow the herb to steep the stronger and more valuable it becomes. Three hours is the maximum time needed to extract the properties fully.

Always keep the pot covered during steeping. After steeping, herbs will fall to the bottom of the pot; so you can either skim off the water, which is now infused with herb principles, or strain it into a jug.

Use only crockery, glass or ceramic pots, or stainless steel or unbroken enamel-lined pans. *Never use aluminium* or *Teflon* pans to steep a herb. For a sage rinse, if you want it to be darker, you may use an iron pan.

Though it is best to take about 3 hours to release the properties of a herb often you won't have that much time. You can use a stainless steel teaspoon, or tea holder, which makes enough for 1 cup. Adjust the recipe accordingly.

Another short cut is to use a coffee infuser. These are made of glass and hold enough for 1 cup. Place 1 or 2 tablespoons of the dried herb in the infuser and pour a cup of boiling water over it. Leave for 15 minutes.

Alternatively, if the herb can be used with milk (as in many facials), *cold* milk absorbs the essences of most herbs *without* heat. Allow 1 tablespoon of the herb to every cup of cold milk. Steep for several hours. Keep the jar covered with a cloth.

Decoction

Decoction is simply boiling. Barks, roots, seeds and chips take at least ½ hour's boiling to release their properties. As with infusions, use stainless steel, crockery or glass only, and remember *to cover the pan* while boiling so as to retain all chemicals and principles released.

Essence

To make an essence, buy an ounce of an essential oil and dissolve in 1 pint of alcohol. Use externally only.

Tincture

Many herbs do not release their properties in water but become active in alcohol (or vinegar). Add 1 ounce of the powdered or crushed herb to 12 ounces* of alcohol, and 4 ounces

---

* When I give liquid quantities in ounces, these are fluid ounces. You can buy a fluid ounce cup or jug which makes measuring much easier.

WAYS OF USING DRIED HERBS

	Kind of Herb	Amount	Liquid
Infusion	most leaves, flowers, herbs use cut instead of powdered	2 tablespoons dried herb	1 pint *boiling* water poured over herb and allowed to steep
Short-cut infusion	most leaves, flowers, herbs	1 tablespoon with *stainless steel* tea ball or spoon	1 cup *boiling* water
Milk infusion	most leaves, flowers, herbs	1 tablespoon	1 cup cold milk will absorb essence of herb when impossible to use heat
Decoction	bark, chips, roots, seeds	2 tablespoons (will expand considerably)	boil herb gently in 1 pint or more water
Essence (use externally only)	oil from herb	1 ounce	dissolve in 1 pint alcohol
Tincture	any powdered or crushed herb	1 ounce	12 ounces alcohol
Extraction	any herb, specially aromatic herb	(1) add as much of herb as will fill ½ cup alcohol without crowding; steep 1 week; strain (2) again add leaves and repeat process	ethanol alcohol
Essential oil	aromatic flowers or leaves	2 tablespoons	oil — either corn, olive, or safflower

WAYS OF USING DRIED HERBS (continued)

Container	Minimum Steeping Time	For Best Results
stainless steel, ceramic, glass; never use Teflon or aluminum; iron okay with sage rinse	leave 3 minutes on heat to 15 minutes off heat; cover pot	3 hours away from heat; cover pot
same as infusion; OR French style coffee infuser which strains off liquid after water absorbs active principles of herb	3 to 5 minutes	
same as infusion	several hours while covered with porous cloth	
same as infusion	20 minutes cover pot	3 hours cover pot
		store in dark place
tight-lidded jar	stand in full sunlight or warm place for 2 weeks	optional — add 1 teaspoon glycerine — store in dark closet
large tight-lidded jar	(1) soak 1 week; pour off leaves; strain through nylon or cheesecloth (2) again add leaves for 1 week and repeat process	· extract is finished when alcohol has characteristic smell of herb. For long lasting extract add: ¼ tsp. tincture of benzoin ¼ tsp. boric acid powder dissolved in 3 tbsp. witch hazel; optional extra ½ tsp. peppermint extract
½ pint bottle filled ¾ full with oil and pounded aromatic herb	3 weeks	closed bottle in full sunlight. Every 7 days strain herbs to obtain clear oil; add fresh pounded herbs; oil is ready when it has strong scent

of water, and place in a tight-lidded jar. Let it stand for 2 weeks either in full sunlight (preferably) or in a warm place. If you like, you can add a teaspoon of glycerine, which nowadays is made from vegetable sources only. Store in a dark cupboard.

Herb Extracts

Infusions and decoctions will not last more than a few days outside of a refrigerator. Therefore when you want to make a herbal preparation longer lasting you will want to know how to prepare an extract. This can be particularly useful with a herbal astringent that uses alcohol.

To ½ cup of alcohol in a jar add as much of a herb as will fill the jar without crowding. Steep for a week and strain. Add more leaves and repeat the same process. After a week pour off the liquid through a nylon or cheesecloth strainer. The extract is finished when the alcohol retains the characteristic smell of the herb.

To make this extract last longer you can add: ¼ teaspoon simple tincture of benzoin, ¼ teaspoon boric acid powder, each of these dissolved in 3 tablespoons of witch hazel. If you wish the extract to have a stronger tingling quality add ½ teaspoon of peppermint extract. Use a tightly lidded jar.

CHAPTER II

SKIN

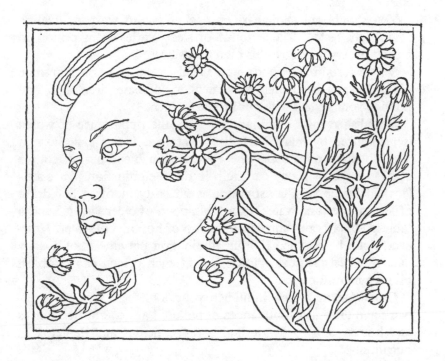

Your skin is one of the miracles of nature, and its perfection should be cherished. It regulates your body temperature, protects you from bacterial invasion and helps you eliminate toxins. If you want your skin to look attractive and healthy there are several rules you must follow. The most important is cleansing with natural and reviving substances, for a clean skin is bound to look healthier. Since constant washing removes most natural oils and moisture, and even the protective acid covering, you must consciously replace these oils, moisture and acid.

Other factors are diet, sleep, exercise and elimination.

Your diet should be high in proteins, which can be found in lean meat, fish and poultry as well as in nuts, beans, milk and eggs. Raw vegetables and fruit of all kinds are essential. Several glasses of water each day are necessary to flush the system clear of toxins.

You should get enough sleep each night to wake up feeling completely rested. The amount of sleep varies from person to person. Everyone knows his own needs best.

Set up a routine of body and facial exercises to fit your time schedule. You need such movement to increase circulation and provide your system with additional oxygen.

Establish regular elimination habits, the importance of which is recognized by many herbalists. Retained toxins can show in poor colour, circles under the eyes or skin blemishes. A couple of figs or prunes a day can help in daily elimination. An excellent aid for chronic constipation is an early morning hot drink of lemon juice and water, or a tablespoon of cider vinegar and a tablespoon of honey stirred into a cup of hot or cool water. However, don't be alarmed if your elimination pattern is not a daily one. The best medical opinion is that each person can establish his own natural pattern.

Other factors which influence your looks are tension, overwork and the outside influences of polluted air, overheated offices and homes, and foods riddled with pesticides and depleted of nutrition.

This chapter is devoted to nutritional aids, cleansing methods, herbal and food solutions to skin problems, and techniques for prevention and eradication of blemishes. A word first about who can use what substances on what kind of skin. People with normal skins (are there any?) may use *any* facial complexion water, soap or wrinkle chaser mentioned in this book. But anyone with oily skin, dry skin, large pores, thread veins or facial and body spot problems should use only those food substances, pharmaceuticals or herbs which are specified in pages dealing with these problems. This chapter also gives herbal and nutritional advice on sunbathing, herbal astringents, cosmetic vinegars and deodorants. Chapter III is devoted to all kinds of baths to restore body moisture, tone and softness. For herbal aids to induce sleep—fatigue being a prime contributor to ageing skin—see Chapter IX.

You will note many references to lanolin in this chapter, indeed in the whole book. Lanolin is the oil washed from the wool of sheep, which resembles our own skin oil, sebum. It is the perfect moisturizer, being not only an emollient but also a humectant (water retainer). There are two kinds of lanolin, hydrous and anhydrous; in this book I always use *anhydrous* lanolin, i.e. lanolin prepared without water, which acts as a better moisturizer, since it can attract water from the air as well as from the deeper levels of the skin. Always ask for *anhydrous* lanolin when buying it.

1. FACIAL EXERCISES

Try not to tense up your facial muscles when you talk and think, and train yourself to relax your face thoroughly whenever you can. Very often you will discover you are keeping certain muscles in a state of constant tension, particularly the muscles around the mouth. Some people even clench or grind their teeth when they are asleep. Once you are aware of this or other grimacing habits you can consciously change them by suddenly relaxing the tensed muscles completely. Do this every time you become aware of the tension, and soon the relaxed state will be natural to you.

You can do the following exercises anywhere—while doing housework, or even while driving (all except the last two). The exercises will have more effect, though, if you massage creams into your face (see page 21), and if you do the exercises lying with your head lower than your feet. Have your palms facing up.

There are four ways to achieve this reversal of gravity. One, of course, is the shoulder stand, the other the unique yoga head-stand—but many people find it difficult to maintain either of these stands. A simple way is to lie with your back on the floor with your feet resting on a bed or sofa. The very best and most relaxing and scientific method of reversal is with a *slant board.* * A folding, cushioned slant board will help you to lie with your head low, and your feet in the air at just the proper angle. Slant boards are an invaluable beauty aid. Whether you take a facial everyday or not, spend at least 15 minutes a day, preferably at the end of the day, on a slant board, for by reversing normal gravity you will tone, re-energize your body and stimulate blood circulation, particularly on your face, which gets very little exercise.

Open your eyes wide and stare to the count of six.

Contract your nose as if you are sneezing and flare out the nostrils.

Lift the side of your mouth to the right as if you were sneering.

Lift the side of your mouth to the left in the same way.

Open the mouth by keeping the upper lip taut and lower lip down.

Purse your lips together as if to whistle.

Open your mouth as if you were going to shout.

Slowly blow up your cheeks and entire upper and lower mouth area and fill with air. Retain air for a count of fifteen and expel with a quick "plop" sound. This gentle exercise will not only help to avoid laugh-line wrinkles, but if done several times a day, might gradually soften existing lines.

With your fists iron your forehead slowly from the middle in an upward sweep to the temples.

With the backs of your outstretched fingers massage your chin from the centre towards the ear in a medium strong patting motion.

For a good double chin exercise, see Section 11.

* Slant boards can be purchased in health food stores, department stores, or through mail order catalogues of Sears, or Hammacher Schlemmer, 147 East Fifty-seventh Street, New York, New York 10022.

2. CLEANSING THE SKIN

You cannot look good unless your face is absolutely clean. The frequency of cleansing should depend on the amount of surface dirt acquired as well as on the oiliness of the skin. Those with an oily skin must clean their face of surface dirt more frequently, as they are more apt to develop blemishes.

There are various methods of cleansing the skin. The first I will mention is steaming, since it can deep-clean the pores. It can be used every day by those with normal and oily skins, and once every 2 weeks by those with dry skin. Other cleansing creams, herbal waters, food scrubs and natural shop soap can be used once a day by those with dry skins, and several times a day by those with oily or normal skin or as specifically indicated.

Whenever possible allow the face to breathe at night free of oils and creams. In this way various accumulated body toxins will be excreted.

Steaming

Many professionals start a deep cleansing of the face with steaming to open the pores and rid of the skin of its impurities. Steam has many uses: it cleanses the skin of surface dirt, stimulates the skin and the circulation, and encourages perspiration, thus helping to get rid of toxins and prevent pimples. For home use I recommend using a simple steam technique or steam combined with a herb infusion. Those with delicate, sensitive skins or those with broken veins on their face *must not use* this technique.

The best face-steaming method with herbs is the foolproof and simple one of pouring boiling water over complexion herbs, improvising a towel-tent, and allowing the steam to soak your face for 10 minutes or more. If you prefer occasionally to use a room vaporizer containing a herb infusion you may do so. But be careful with the directed steam from the vaporizer. Don't go out for at least an hour after you have opened your pores in this manner, and be sure to close the pores once they are clean.

Different herbs have different properties. Some aid in the cleansing process, some increase circulation, others remove impurities, still others are wrinkle-preventers. A few have the capacity to heal rough skin and lesions. Others tighten and stimulate. Some of these herbs also prevent and control blemishes.

The following herbs can be used for steaming, individually or in combination. Note that these same herbs can be used in facials (see Section 4).

versatile

chamomile
elder flower

cleansing, neutral, soothing

chamomile (also good with
    thyme and lavender)

removes impurities

fennel
nettle
lime flowers (linden)
hay flower
oat flowers

drying/astringent

yarrow
lady's mantle

cleansing/circulation boosters

nettle
rosemary

stimulating/tightening

peppermint
elder flower
simple tincture of benzoin
balsam of Gilead
gum tragacanth
gum arabic
horsetail

healing

houseleek
comfrey
fennel

For specific blemish prevention herbs see Section 5.

How to Remove Blackheads after Steaming

You can remove most blackheads and whiteheads after plain or herbal steaming by pushing gently with a tissue or a cotton swab in a gently rotating circle. You will make your task easier by using a make-up mirror with side lights. For the really difficult-to-remove blackheads and whiteheads or other blemishes, see Section 5.

Once you have removed the white- or blackheads, close your pores with such astringents as chamomile or lady's mantle infusion, or peeled cucumber, lemon juice and water, rose water or witch hazel. There is a full description of food and herbal astringents in Section 13. If you have no astringents immediately available you can use cool water, or in the case of normal and oily skin, a piece of ice. However, those with thin skin or thread veins must never subject their skin to extreme temperatures.

Cleansing Cream

Cleansing cream is one of the oldest complexion-care products. It was developed nearly two thousand years ago by the Greek physician Galen who combined olive oil, wax and rose water. My version is a variation with sweet almond oil (or avocado oil). This is a simple recipe with the purest ingredients; it costs very little and is the equivalent of the most expensive cream on the market.

white wax	½ ounce
anhydrous lanolin	1 ounce
sweet almond oil (or avocado)	3 ounces
rose water	1 ounce

optional

several drops of flower oil or essence (do not use if allergic)

Melt the white wax and lanolin in a double boiler. Slowly add the almond oil and blend in the rose water, stirring all the time. Remove from the heat. Add aromatic oil or essence (optional). Pour into labelled opaque jar.

Cocoa butter is another exceptional cleanser for the skin. Not only is it nourishing for the face, neck and hands, but it has a delightful smell.

You can make a cocoa butter cleansing liquid as follows:

cocoa butter	1 tablespoon
anhydrous lanolin	1 tablespoon
avocado oil (or sweet almond oil or safflower oil)	½ cup

In the top of a double boiler, melt together the cocoa butter, the lanolin and avocado oil until they are all completely dissolved and blended together. Beat with an electric mixer until the combination is slightly cooled. Pour into labelled jar. Shake before using.

To adapt this recipe for dry skin, to every 3 tablespoons of the cocoa butter cleansing liquid, add 1 tablespoon of water. This will give you the added moisture-content dry skin needs. Pour into a labelled jar. Shake vigorously before using. For other dry skin advice see Sections 3, 4 and 8.

Herbal Cleansing Waters

Many herbs, either in infusion or in distilled form, help clean the face. They also have healing and soothing powers. You can make these infusions and use them strained, but they do not last long unless you keep them in the refrigerator. For this reason it is useful to be able to buy distilled herbal waters; the Society of Herbalists have an excellent distilled elder flower water in Caswell-Massey in New York and the Culpeper shops in London.

Elder flower water was once considered an absolute necessity for the complexion, and earlier generations relied on it to keep the skin fair and free of blemishes. It has not lost its reputation among present-day herbalists. The French call it *eau de sureau* and consider it stimulating, cleansing and mildly astringent. Old herbals sometimes call it *aqua sambuci*.

I learned the following recipe from my Rumanian grandmother who told me it went back many generations in our family:

buttermilk	½ pint
elder blossoms	5 tablespoons
honey	2 tablespoons

Gently heat the buttermilk and soak the elder blossoms in it. Keep warm and simmering for ½ hour until the blossoms soften. Remove from heat. Steep for 3 hours. Reheat. Strain. Add honey. Keep refrigerated. Use as a face cleanser.

Elder blossoms can also be used in your bath water to soften your skin (see Chapter III).

A recipe for *virgin milk,* with variations and under different names, often appears in old herbals and books of cosmetic lore. Why was it called virgin (sometimes virginal) milk? Possibly because a glass of water becomes pure milky white instantaneously when the tincture of benzoin is added; or because it has such a clearing effect on the skin. Used as a cleanser it will soften and soothe the skin, and it is also an old English remedy for pimples and red spots:

| simple† tincture of benzoin | 15 drops |
| glass of water (spring or distilled if possible) | |

optional

| glycerine | 3 drops |
| tincture of myrrh | 3 drops |

Instead of water you can use rose, orange or elder flower water. In Chapter X you will find an inexpensive recipe for homemade rose and orange water.

A strong infusion of dried pimpernel flowers, *pimpernel water,* may be kept in the refrigerator and used daily as an astringent complexion cleanser. This was another well-known standby, and references to it even appear in Restoration comedy: "Oh, why

† Use only simple tincture, not compound tincture. The compound has elements added which are harmful to the skin. If your chemist doesn't stock it, ask him to order some, or make some up for you.

does she have such a huge freckle on her face? She should use my pimpernel water!"

Plantain water is another herbal cleanser. Plantain is one of the commonest garden weeds and can be found on most lawns. The Greeks considered it a healing herb. In the Highlands they call it by the Gaelic word "slanlus" which means "plant of healing." The crushed leaves can be applied directly for many skin problems, bites, stings, swellings and bruises. Several ancient herbalist sources mention plantain in combination with other cosmetic healing items such as houseleek and lemon juice, or as Mrs. Hagger recorded under "Severall Select Experiments," plantain water mixed with pounded almonds. To make plantain water, add boiling water to the fresh washed leaves and steep for ½ hour or longer. Strain. Refrigerate.

Food Cleansers

A *sunflower seed cleanser,* rich in natural vitamin E and lecithin, is simple to make in small or large quantities. Grind, or blend, 2 tablespoons of sunflower seed kernels to 1 teaspoon of water (preferably distilled or pure mineral water). If you like to experiment, add a scant ¼ teaspoon of honey and ¼ teaspoon of sunflower oil. This will give you a smoother effect, but will be slightly sticky because of the honey.

Normal and oily skin food cleansers. For cleansing normal or oily skin, peeled or grated potato is particularly good. It has been used for centuries to cleanse the skin of impurities and blemishes. It has been claimed to cure eczema. Potato water wash is made by extracting the juice in a vegetable juicer. Make it fresh each day, or keep a large amount in a labelled jar in your refrigerator. Potatoes are healing, cleansing and nourishing for the skin.

Yogurt plus a few grains of salt can also be used by those with oily and normal skin (see Section 6).

Dry skin must be cleansed in a special way. Do not use ordinary soaps, as although they will remove grime, they contribute to the dry condition. Almond oil and avocado oil are excellent cleansers for those with dry skin. Earlier in this section (page

14) is a special cocoa butter dry skin liquid cleanser. Natural soaps, glycerine soaps, vegetable soaps and super fatted oatmeal soaps are suitable cleansers. For additional facts on dry skin see Section 8.

Oatmeal, almond meal, cornmeal and bran are still in everyday use in many parts of the world as a substitute for soap. In parts of India, a form of cornmeal is used for complexion scrub material and as a cleansing powder, and is brushed through the hair. These meals are all valuable assets in complexion care, since they contain vegetable hormones which nourish the skin.

Any of these meals can be put into a small lidded jar and kept in the bathroom. They are effective with water added to them. For a stronger body scrub, they can be used with a rough flannel or loofah. In my home we prefer colloidal oatmeal, a suspended particle version of oatmeal, which dissolves easily and leaves the skin with a creamy, silky texture. Those with allergic or adolescent skin will find it efficacious as a body, face and hand "soap."

Lemon is such an obvious cleanser that most people have forgotten about it. But it is truly effective, particularly on the hands, and will overcome any strong food odours such as fish or garlic. Since it gets mouldy, keep only small amounts in the kitchen or bathroom.

While I was travelling in the west of England, an enchanting lady told me her family lemon-cleansing recipe:

> whole lemon
> rock candy‡   several pieces
> gold leaf or aluminium foil
> hot ashes

Make a hole in a lemon. Fill the inside with rock candy, and close the cavity with gold leaf or aluminium foil. Roast the lemon in the hot ashes of a fireplace, or use charcoal brickets in a hibachi barbecue. When you need lemon juice, squeeze out a little through a hole in the gold leaf or foil on to a cloth and wash your face.

‡ Rock candy, pieces of sugar on a string, is used for coughs and is available from old-fashioned chemists.

She had an exceptionally good complexion and she claimed that the juice not only cleansed her face but brightened it.

Soap

Of all the commercial soaps I prefer those which include glycerine. *Pears* is such a soap. This pure product, which can still be bought in every chemist's, goes back many years. A nineteenth-century toiletry book, by Anna Kingsford, quotes a leading dermatologist of the time as follows. "The more nearly negative a soap is, the nearer does it approach perfection. It is essentially in this respect that *Pears* soap excels. I have reason to think that *Pears* soap is the best because it is the purest ever made, an opinion vouched for by the strictness of chemical analysis. So effectually for medical purposes has the process of purification been carried out, that this soap when made up in a lather, can be applied to the surface abraded by eczema."

By a "negative" soap she means a soap with as little alkaline content as possible—though it has to have some, or it would not be soap. Fairly neutral negative soaps are made from oatmeal and vegetables, and plants such as aloes and amole. These can be bought at some chemists or health food stores.

Since most home soaps are made with lye, no such recipes are included in this book. If you know of a recipe without lye, and would like to share it, please contact me through the publisher.

Hundreds of growing things contain saponin, a natural soaping ingredient, found in various leaves, flowers, twigs, bulbs, berries and trees.

The best known, and my favourite soap source, is one called by many names, including soapwort. "Wort" is the old English word for plant or herb, and is often found as the final syllable in country names for herbs, particularly those with a medicinal or superstitious application. Soapwort is also known as bouncing Bet, and while it was once a cultivated garden plant only, it now grows wild and can be found in profusion in wastelands. In the American South it is sometimes called my lady's washbowl. It was known to European peasants, and was often used by mediaeval monks, who called it fuller's herb.

Bouncing Bet or soapwort is a perennial which blooms along roadsides and meadows from July to September. It is a very pretty plant about 2 feet tall with 1-inch pink (sometimes white) flowers which grow in loose clusters. Although the stems contain a gummy juice which will produce a lather, it is the root which is mucilaginous and soapy when agitated in water.

Yucca, Chlorogalum, Lamb's Quarters

These three soapy plants are American Indian discoveries. All are excellent for skin care, or hair shampooing and clothes washing.

Yucca or Spanish bayonet is a striking cultivated plant with spiky, rigid leaves. It also grows wild in the southwest United States, particularly in New Mexico and Arizona. It is called amole in parts of Mexico and there are several amole soaps on the market. Soap made from yucca is most agreeable to the skin, for it leaves it soft, and is useful for clothes washing as well as hair shampoos.

The rootstock of yucca is rather deep, so you might need a crowbar to uproot it. Use this soap root by breaking into little pieces and washing free of dirt and grit. It can be activated directly in water or in a muslin bag.

Chlorogalum (*pomeridianum*) is a part of the lily family and grows wild in the hilly sections of California. To discover this bulb look in the late spring for a cluster of stemless, grass-like leaves that later form into a tall spray of widely spread, white, small, lily-like blossoms. These emerge a few at a time in the evening and wither by the next day.

The bulb when dug out looks like a coconut husk light bulb. Strip the hairy, fibrous coat to find the moist heart 1 or 2 inches wide and 2 to 4 inches long. Crush this *inner* bulb and rub it briskly in water for a wonderful non-alkali shampoo that leaves the hair soft and glossy and eliminates dandruff. This soap can be dried and used many months later.

Lamb's quarters or pigweed is a weedy-looking plant with

greenish flowers and triangular leaves which turn yellow. The fresh root is deep, spindle-shaped and quite brittle. It is easily crushed into soap form when agitated in water.

Pacific coast *lilac, myrtle, buckbush* are another source of excellent soap. These fresh blossoms provide the rarest of treats—a sort of Polynesian island fantasy good for cleansing and for skin softening.

Be careful when picking these flowers not to pick also the green stalks or you will have a green lather with a funny smell. The green seed vessels can also be used as a soap, but if not rinsed right off leave a yellow stain.

There are three species of tree that have small white flowers and fleshy berries about the size of cherries, which in turn contain one or two seeds that lather in water. I offer the Latin names so that they can be looked up in a tree book. *Sapindus saponaria* can be found on the tip of Florida; *S. marginatus* is an evergreen found along the Atlantic seaboard from the Carolinas to Florida; *S. drummandi* is to be found from Kansas to Louisiana and westward to Arizona. This tree is also called soapberry or wild China tree, as it resembles the true China tree, or jaboncillo (little soap). This tree has clusters of yellow berries, which turn black as they dry and can readily be seen in the bare winter winds until spring.

Those of you who beachcomb should look for the small yellowish split-pea size *eggs* of the *sea snail* as they are excellent washballs. A sailor friend tells me that many old fishermen and sailors prefer these eggs to ordinary store-bought soap.

3. WRINKLES

Any number of things can cause or prevent wrinkles. Not that some wrinkles aren't on the positive side—especially the ones that come from lots of laughter and smiles. Certain crinkles in fact give personality to the face. But deep, ridged wrinkles and parchment skin often come from factors you can control, such as lack of moisture and oils, constant grimacing, or loss of tone and elasticity resulting from lack of protein. To give your skin tone you must eat protein, for otherwise the body uses up its stored protein and the muscles sag, and folds and wrinkles appear. Other internal nourishers are foods with vitamins A, B complex, C, D and E. You also need lots of fresh water and body and facial exercises to keep your face youthful. For other wrinkle-prevention techniques see this chapter, Sections 4, 8 and 11; Chapter V, Section 32; and the facial exercises at the beginning of this chapter.

Massage Techniques for Applying Creams

Massage the neck and under the chin with upward, outward motions.

Massage the chin area with upward motions, forward and over the jawline towards the ears.

Massage laugh lines upwards, over the upper cheek towards the outer section of the eye.

Delicately pat the under-eye area from nose bridge out to temples.

Gently massage crows feet upwards towards the temples.

Massage the forehead from the middle. Stroke upwards with two hands each going in upward, outward motions towards opposite upper temples.

Wrinkle-chaser Food—Internal

Brewer's yeast, taken internally in tablet, powder or flake form, can help you avoid and gradually overcome heavy creases and folds in the skin.

Take 2 tablespoons a day. People sometimes find they feel "gassy" with yeast. This means the body really needs it. The feeling will eventually go away when the body requirements for these nutrients are met. To overcome the feeling of gassiness, you can take coated hydrochloric acid pills, which will quickly adjust the gas reaction.

Lanolin and Vitamin E Moisturizer

Vitamin E has many internal uses and is also efficacious in first aid for cuts and burns, but few people know that it is very useful as a skin moisturizer. It can be used alone, but is rather thick and slightly sticky when it comes out of the capsule. A few drops of anhydrous lanolin (or glycerine) give it a better consistency. For the skin it doesn't matter what kind of vitamin E you use—the E complex should be perfectly suitable. Taken internally, vitamin E increases circulation, and is therefore excellent for the skin.

Vitamin Nourishing Cream

This is my favourite nourishing cream since it contains both vitamin E and vitamin A. These two vitamins are an inexpensive and indispensable addition to your toiletry shelf. Vitamin E is sold in International Units (I.U.); vitamin A in units BP. Vitamin E tends to be expensive, so you may want to use less. I give the maximum amount in parentheses.

The cream should be used after you have cleansed your skin, as a skin *food*. Try to use the cream, if possible, an hour or two before you go to bed. Then wipe it off gently. Whenever possible your skin should be allowed to breathe, free of creams, when you sleep.

beeswax	1½ tablespoons
white wax	1 tablespoon
anhydrous lanolin	1 tablespoon (liquid or solid)
sweet almond oil	3 ounces (avocado oil or safflower oil can also be used)
distilled water	1 ounce
borax	½ teaspoon
rose water	1 ounce (instead of distilled water you can use 2 ounces of rose water)

simple tincture of benzoin (not compound)
2 to 6 capsules of vitamin E (400 I.U.)
2 to 6 capsules of vitamin A (25,000 units)

In a double boiler, heat together the beeswax, the white wax and the lanolin. Slowly add almond, avocado or safflower oil. In a separate pan (glass or stainless steel) heat 1 ounce of distilled water; and the borax (this acts as a special emulsifier) until the borax dissolves completely. Slowly add the rose water so that it too is slightly warm. Now without allowing either pan to get cool, add the rose water and borax combination to the wax, lanolin and oil combination and beat with an electric beater for as long as it takes for the cream to cool to room temperature. Add the simple tincture of benzoin. Prick open your vitamin capsules, add to cream and beat until the vitamins are blended.

For a nourishing eye cream see Chapter V.

Lily Root and Lanolin Cream Nourisher

Lily and narcissus roots have formidable reputations in complexion and wrinkle care. Use them pulverized with other complexion herbs, honey and rose water to make a complexion water. Make sure they are insecticide free.

water	1 cup
powdered lily roots	2 tablespoons
honey	1 tablespoon
anhydrous lanolin	1 ounce
rose water	½ teaspoon

Add a cup of water to powdered lily root. Simmer in covered pot for ½ hour. Strain and add honey. To make into cream, add an ounce of liquid or solid lanolin melted in a double boiler. Add rose water. Put into a labelled jar.

Avocado Cream Skin Nourisher

whole eggs	2
glycerine	1 teaspoon
lemon juice	½ teaspoon
avocado oil	enough to thicken mixture
sea salt	pinch
cider vinegar	⅛ teaspoon
egg yolks	3
water (or orange or rose)	2 tablespoons

optional

vitamin A	50,000 units
vitamin E	400 I.U.

Blend together fresh eggs, glycerine, lemon juice. Slowly add drop by drop enough avocado oil to thicken the mixture. Add sea salt, cider vinegar. When this is thickened to a cream-like consistency add beaten egg yolks and the water. Completely blend the mixture. Pour into a labelled jar. This must be kept in a refrigerator.

Sweet Cream Line-eraser

Sweet cream is a nourishing food for the complexion. Always remember to pat it on in the manner described under massage techniques.

Onto a thoroughly clean skin pat a mixture of a whipped egg white and a teaspoon of cream. Allow to dry for 20 minutes and wash off with tepid water.

Myrrh Facial

Athenian ladies used this wrinkle-prevention facial. It was made by burning powdered myrrh, a powerful healing astringent resin, in an iron plate, allowing the fumes to penetrate the skin of the face as if using a steam sauna. Myrrh is available from some chemists and botanical sources.

Onion Water

Fresh onions are reputedly marvellous for the skin and can prevent blemishes. Mash, blend or pulverize the onion and use the juice. According to many ancient herbalists, the juice can also be added to honey and white wax and used as an anti-wrinkle preparation.

Eau de Circe

Circe was the sorceress described by Homer, who turned the companions of Odysseus into swine. Over the years her name has come to be applied to any fascinating or irresistible woman.

In an ancient French toiletry book I found the following recipe for "Eau de Circe." The French considered it an aid in preventing wrinkles. The gum benzoin and the alcohol will tighten and dry the skin, so don't use the preparation if you have dry skin.

ethyl alcohol (70%)	8 ounces
simple tincture of benzoin	4 drops
melted gum arabic	4 drops
oil of sweet almonds	1 drop
pulverized ground cloves	pinch
ground nutmeg	pinch
rose water	1½ ounces

Pour the alcohol into a clean quart bottle. Add the benzoin, gum arabic, oil of sweet almonds and the cloves and nutmeg. Shake together. Let the preparation stand for a few days, shaking it occasionally; then add rose water. Use it at night before retiring.

4. FACIALS

The aim of a facial mask is to clean, restore, nourish and awaken the skin. The outcome should be a downy, smoother, fresher face. Dozens of simple home products can be used in facials, including healing and skin-restoring household items like honey, milk, yogurt, buttermilk, whey, egg white, egg yolk, lemon, vinegar, hormone-rich cereal and nut meals, vegetable, animal and nut oils, fruits and vegetables, as well as herbal and clay products.

You can experiment by mixing together any of the substances mentioned in this section—unless you have oily or dry skin, in which case note carefully which of the ingredients mentioned are good for your type of skin, and check in Sections 6 and 8, where you will find facials for your specific problem. If your mixture comes out too runny, use the following binding substances: banana, honey, fuller's earth, kaolin, almond meal, oatmeal, whole egg; egg yolk for dry skin, egg white, yogurt or buttermilk for oily skin.

Ingredients for Facials

Two neutral facial *clays* which are often mentioned are kaolin and fuller's earth. They can be added to any mask to give more body and firmness. Fuller's earth is an absorbent clay which was originally used by fullers, in cloth mills, to remove grease from fabrics, when the cloth was being cleaned and thickened for the market. (It is also mentioned elsewhere in this book as a dusting powder for feet, and as a dry shampoo for the hair.) Kaolin is the fine white clay used in the manufacture of porcelain.

Yet another useful inert clay for masks is bentonite. Because it is healing and soothing it is sometimes used by dermatologists for treatment of wounds, sores and eczema.

The *milk and egg products* suggested for facials each have

particular uses. Please note the restrictions on all these products; they depend on the quality and texture of your skin. People with normal and youthful skin can use *any* milk or lactic acid milk product, or egg white, egg yolk or whole egg in their facial masks. People with dry skin should only use the lecithin rich* egg yolk in masks, since egg white is too drying. Dry-skinned people must also restrict their milk soothers, healers and binders to sour cream, sweet cream, skim milk and whole milk. Those with oily skin will learn to appreciate the drying, tightening qualities of beaten egg white, whey and the lactic acid products, buttermilk and yogurt.

Of the many *oils* which can be used as facial nourishers, wheat germ oil, avocado oil and almond oil are preferred. However, you can substitute wheat germ flour, crushed whole avocado, powder from pulverized almonds or the grocery shop emollients, safflower, peanut, corn or olive oil.

Gum resins such as benzoin, tragacanth and arabic are most useful as tightening agents. Benzoin is also a skin cleanser, and can be used in dozens of different facials and creams. Benzoin is soluble in alcohol. To learn how to make an alcohol tincture, see Chapter I. Gum tragacanth is soluble by leaving in water for 24 hours—the ribbon variety dissolves more easily; gum arabic, which comes from Africa, can be dissolved in double its weight of water.

Vegetables and fruits contain a myriad trace minerals, many enzymes and vitamins. Some have an acid effect on the skin, some are neutral and others are alkaline.

The skin has a certain amount of acidity, called an acid mantle. The pH value is a way of expressing acidity and alkalinity on a scale from 0 to 14; the skin has a value between 4 and 6, generally taken as 5.5. The acid mantle acts as a protective barrier against infection. A healthy skin produces its own acid mantle within a few hours of washing, but constant washing or swimming can be destructive, and you can help replace the acidity with judicious use of various food products patted on the skin. This is why cider vinegar is such a useful skin aid. Cider

* Lecithin, an invaluable skin aid, can also be obtained in liquid form.

vinegar can be drying used undiluted, but used diluted as it would be in a bath it is good for any texture skin and helps normalize it.

The most neutral of the fruits and vegetables are the cucumber, watermelon, fig, raw horse-radish, onion, persimmon, sweet green pepper and banana. Tomato is not very acid. The least acid foods, which will be a great help to people with dry skin, are cantaloupe, avocado, honeydew melon, olive, lettuce, carrot. If you need an acid boost to the skin, these are the most acid foods you can use in a facial, starting with the highest acidity: lime, lemon, grapes, cranberry, strawberry, pineapple, grapefruit, apple.

You can use any of the above foods squeezed or patted on the face as you're preparing them to eat. Allow them to dry on the face and wash off with tepid water. If you want a more formal facial, mash up 2 tablespoons of any of the above foods and mix with a binder: honey is a neutral binder; buttermilk, yogurt, clays, earth, egg white are drying binders good for oily skin; banana, sour cream and egg yolk are good binders for dry skin. Always add 5 or 6 drops of cider vinegar; or try adding a dollop of your favourite oil and 2 or 3 drops of cider vinegar to a dry skin facial.

Other ingredients. Lanolin is a good ingredient for facials, as it is water-attracting. Glycerine has the same qualities. Honey is another water-attracting product and is extremely healing and nourishing for the skin. Buy uncooked honey whenever possible, and use it for creams, facials and special baths as well as instead of sugar.

Cider vinegar can be added to almost any mask. Brewer's yeast can be used in a facial (see Sections 6 and 8 for other uses).

Herbs for Facials

Many herbs are useful for facials. Fennel, nettle, oat flowers, hay flower and lime flowers (linden) can help release impurities from the skin. Use them in the pre-facial steaming. Other skin-cleansing herbs are the mild and apple-fragrant chamomile, and lady's mantle. Nettle and rosemary will increase the circulation. Elder flower, horse tail and peppermint are stimulating and tightening for the skin. The best herbs for oily skin are lady's mantle and the very astringent yarrow. When the skin is damaged from too much sun or an infection or wound, use healing herbs such as fennel, houseleek, marshmallow and comfrey. Comfrey has always been known as a wound healer and is used as an internal healer in Russia; it contains allantoin, which seems to stimulate skin cell growth. The Doubleday Foundation of England is investigating ways of using this valuable herb.

Irish moss, quince seed and flaxseed will also soften the skin. Soften the herb in hot water, allow to cool, and add to the facial. These gelatinous herbs are useful for clay masks which harden on the face, as the mask will come off in one piece.

Blemish-controlling herbs are listed separately in Section 5; use any of these in facials.

How to Use Herbs in Facials

All the herbs mentioned may be used in infusion unless otherwise noted. Pour a pint of boiling water over 2 tablespoons, steep for 15 minutes to 3 hours and strain. Use only *1* tablespoon of the herb infusion in the facial; keep the rest for a face wash, or for any of the many other uses most herbs have. Put it in a labelled jar in the refrigerator.

Comfrey contains a great deal of mucilage, which is softening and healing. You can use comfrey by infusing the leaves and adding it to a steam facial; by mashing the fresh leaves and using it as a compress on the face, or by boiling ½ ounce of the crushed root in 1 *quart* of milk or water. Strain and add a tablespoon of either the infusion or the decoction to any facial.

An infusion can be made from dried fennel fruit; or a decoction from the seed. Use dried houseleek leaves in infusion, or pound fresh houseleek in a marble mortar and squeeze out the juice; pour a few drops of ethyl alcohol or vodka on the juice when you want to use it. It will turn milky.

How to Use a Facial Mask

First cleanse the skin. For a thoroughly deep pore-cleansing before a facial, first steam your face as described in Section 2. If you steam your face, or are going to use a clay or earth mask, or an almond meal or oatmeal mask, which absorb dirt from the pores, you do *not* have to cleanse the skin with a complexion water or cream.

Gently pat the mixed ingredients on to your face. Allow between 15 and 30 minutes for the mask to "take." You can intensify the effect of a mask by lying down quietly with herb-soaked pads covering the eyes, and with your feet higher than your head. Afterwards wash off the mask with cotton wool or a soft face flannel and tepid water. Make sure that the hairline and ears are clean. The pores will be wide open, so close them with a gentle astringent (see Section 13).

Often you will have more than you need for one facial. Some ingredients can be stored in the refrigerator for the next day, but eggs coagulate and many other items harden when mixed together, so you are better off using leftovers immediately as a hand or body rub. Some facial masks make excellent healing and restoring body lotions. They are particularly effective on areas which sometimes have dead skin: the buttocks, and elbows and the backs of the legs.

Honey Circulation Facials

Honey is a remarkably versatile natural product. It acts as a *moisturizing* agent and is therefore particularly good for dry skin. It is also *stimulating, soothing* and *healing.* It can be applied to roughened skin blemishes—alone or in combination with many other natural substances. If you wish, you can add a tablespoon to any facial listed in this book.

The following ingredients mix especially well with honey:

Pulverized almonds, almond oil, almonds and milk.
Avocado, wheat germ, safflower, sesame, peanut, corn oil.

For normal or oily skin: beaten egg white, or egg white and ¼ teaspoon of either lemon or cider vinegar.

For dry skin: egg yolk, a few drops of cider vinegar, any of the oils mentioned above.

Any complexion herb.

Moisturizing Facials

Every skin can benefit from a moisturizing boost, particularly since sunshine, polluted air and dry centrally heated indoor air removes much of the moisture from the skin.

One of the best moisturizers is vitamin E. Prick a capsule of 100 I.U. (International Units) of this vitamin and smear it on your face as often as possible. Since it is rather thick, try to mix it with a little liquefied anhydrous lanolin.

Glycerine is a moisturizer which will extract water from lower tissues of the skin and from the air. You can use glycerine with rose water.

Honey and peach juice are also moisturizers.

Use any of these products in conjunction with such penetrating oils as avocado, wheat germ or almond. Or use safflower, olive or corn oil in your facials.

In making a mask with these materials add any or all of the following ingredients: egg white or egg yolk, or milk products such as sour cream, yogurt, buttermilk, milk, sweet cream, clay products.

Moisturizer-lotion Mask

This combination of oils and vitamins will sink into your skin and leave it feeling refreshed, soft and moist. It will feed the skin and by helping to keep it elastic prevent the onset of wrinkles. You can occasionally leave the mask on overnight, but not often, as your facial pores should breathe freely while you sleep.

The mask relies on several healing oils and two skin-nourishing vitamins—A and E. Since these are all stable oils you can double or triple the recipe. Use a dark bottle if you can, and be sure to label the contents.

Figures in parentheses are maximum quantities.

wheat germ oil	1 tablespoon
avocado oil	2 tablespoons
almond oil	1 tablespoon
sesame oil†	2 tablespoons
vitamin A‡	2 capsules (50,000 units)
vitamin E	2 capsules (400 I.U.)

Mix oils together. Prick open capsules and add to oils. Shake vigorously. Label jar. To make a harder mask add clay, honey, egg or a milk product.

Deep Pore Cleansing Clay Mask

beeswax	⅛ ounce
lanolin (anhydrous)	1 ounce
rose water	⅛ pint
fuller's earth	4 ounces

optional

teaspoon of melted quince seed, flax seed (linseed), or Irish moss (carragheen), or teaspoon of unflavoured dissolved gelatine: vegetable colouring

This is a famous salon facial mask, one which they charge a lot of money for. The lanolin is a marvellous emollient. The fuller's earth will absorb dirt.

Melt the wax, together with the lanolin, in a double boiler.

---

† Do not buy the dark Japanese sesame oil as it smells too strong.
‡ Vitamin A is usually made from a fish oil. For a non-fishy odour use one made from palm oil or lemon grass.

Add the rose water and stir thoroughly. Add the vegetable colouring if you want to tint the mask. If you like a scented mask this is the time to add a few drops of your favourite essence or cologne. Stir in the fuller's earth and work all in a mortar until a smooth mixture is obtained.

You can double or triple the quantities in this recipe to make a long-lasting larger batch.

The Spring Peeler Facial

This is a once-in-a-while facial for after the winter, or after an illness or high fever when your face looks sallow and saggy.

Rub your favourite vegetable or nut oil (such as wheat germ oil, avocado oil, almond oil) over your entire face and neck. Immediately pat on gently a drop of warm water and over that pat on a third layer of pure lemon juice (if possible). Wait for about a minute, but not long enough for the oil or lemon to dry.

With your index and middle finger start rubbing this emulsion with a circular motion until a little ball forms. Discard the ball and collect another ball until your face looks fresh and peeled.

Papaya Peeler

A steam infusion of papaya tea, or application of papaya juice, will remove dead skin cells from the face. Papaya contains an enzyme which can soften protein tissue. Do not rub it into the skin, as the action of this fruit is quite strong. After steaming, gently wash the face with tepid water and close pores with a mild astringent. If you are using papaya juice straight on the face, wash off after 5 minutes, dry face with a soft cloth, and close pores with a mild astringent.

Pre-party Facials and Masks

Women have been using mud and food on their faces for thousands of years, and I delight in this quotation from the Roman poet Juvenal, who complains that the Roman husband hardly ever recognizes his wife while she is at home because of her masks, and it is only when she sallies forth to the market, festival or party that:

> The eclipse then vanishes, and all her face
> Is open'd and restored to every grace
> The crust removed, her cheeks as smooth as silk
> Are polish'd with a wash of asses milk.

What you want before a party is something to nourish the skin and increase the circulation of your face so that you look particularly bright and glowing. There are many products which can brighten, tingle and enliven the skin temporarily.

Egg white tightener. Beat 1 egg white and pat on face. It will tighten immediately. Allow to dry for 15 minutes and rinse off with tepid water and cotton wool.

Cinderella make-up tightener. This is a make-up secret told me by my husband, a film make-up man. Technically it is not a facial mask but rather a partial facial left on under make-up. It is an under-eye tightener, and is useful for a special party, a photography session or a day when you don't feel at your best and want to look extra special. But alas, as with Cinderella you must leave "the ball" after a few hours, for the tightener only lasts that long.

egg white	¼

Beat egg white until frothy. With a thin brush (Japanese writing brushes from artists' suppliers are perfect) paint a very, very thin paste of the egg white under the eyes. The area will tighten. Pat a liquid make-up over the egg white.

Tincture of benzoin circulation booster. This is a cleansing, softening and tightening mask which will make your face tingle and feel more alive.

simple tincture of benzoin	½ teaspoon
glycerine	½ teaspoon
rose water	½ teaspoon
fuller's earth or kaolin	2 ounces

Make a paste of all ingredients. Pat on face with fingers or cotton. Allow the mask to harden for 15 to 30 minutes. Wash off with warm water. Close pores with a mild astringent.

Pre-party mask. Many of the resins from trees can be melted and used as skin tighteners. These are stimulating and may also bring out impurities from the system. For this reason the mask should be used two days before the party.

You can use gum tragacanth, gum benzoin (or simple tincture of benzoin) or balsam of Gilead. Melt the gum and mix together with a tablespoon of anhydrous lanolin. Allow the mask to dry for 15 minutes, and wash off with tepid water. Avoid the area near the eyes.

Cereal healing masks. Various cereals have a whitening, softening, soothing effect on the skin. Apply to face or any rough spots on your body.

Use 1 tablespoon of almond paste, almond oil, oatmeal paste or colloidal oatmeal. Blend in a teaspoon of milk, apple pulp, honey or egg yolk. Apply to the face with a patting motion.

Mask for puffy face. There are many anti-inflammatory herbs. Chamomile or lady's mantle infusion can be used in a compress, or these same herbs can be added to stiffly beaten egg whites and patted on the face. A stiffly beaten egg white alone can be used to reduce puffiness. A 5-minute mask should be sufficient.

Russian mask. A modernized version of a mask favoured by Russian ladies consists of a tablespoon of healing wheat germ oil, a whipped egg yolk, and a few drops of cider vinegar. Pat on face. Allow to dry for 15 minutes. Wash off with tepid water.

Allergic Skin Facial

wheat germ oil (or flour)	1 tablespoon
yogurt	1 tablespoon

Mix the oil (or flour) and yogurt together until smooth. Pat on face and neck. Allow to dry for 15 minutes. Remove gently with a large, smooth towel or with cotton wool dipped in tepid water. Close pores with an astringent such as rose water or cucumber. Never rub sensitive skin.

Anti-wrinkle Facials

No amount of herb facials will be effective for wrinkles without the right diet (see Section 3). But herbs can soften and lubricate the skin, and help in cell regeneration.

Four herbs in particular—comfrey, fennel, houseleek and marshmallow—have been used for centuries both as healing herbs and in the fight against the encroachment of time. See *How to Use Herbs in Facials* (page 29) for ways of using comfrey, fennel and houseleek.

Houseleek is a fibrous root herb which grows on the walls of houses and even on the roofs. In the past it was used as an instant first aid. The juices from the leaves were used to cure scalds and heal sores. It was the favourite herb of Ninon de Lenclos, the renowned French beauty and wit who was born in 1620 and died in 1705 still beautiful. Her nightly facial consisted of the expressed juice of fresh houseleek added to lanolin and almond oil. It is also an excellent herb for skin inflammations and a treasured remedy for pimples. The Greek physician Galen recommended houseleek even for erysipelas and shingles. You can add the juice of the houseleek to any nourishing ointment.

Marshmallow is another herb with softening agents. The dried roots, boiled in water, give out half their weight of a gummy substance similar to starch. Or you can soak an ounce of the roots in cold water for half an hour and then peel off the bark, cut up the root, and soak for a few more hours.

The Duchess of Alba Anti-wrinkle Facial

The handsome Duchess of Alba left some interesting stories about her life and loves, as well as an eternal record of her beauty in Goya's painting.

According to the diary which contained this recipe, it could be used as both a facial and a night mask. "This will not only keep out the wrinkles and preserve the complexion fair, but it is a great remedy where the skin becomes too loosely attached to the muscles, as it gives firmness to the parts." However, although this is an anti-wrinkle mask, the alum and egg white are tightening and drying, so it is more suitable for oily skin than for those with a tendency towards dry skin.

egg whites	4
rose water	to cover
alum powder	½ ounce
oil of sweet almonds	¼ ounce

Beat egg whites and boil in the rose water. Add alum and almond oil. Beat all these ingredients together until they assume the consistency of a paste.

Vegetable and Fruit Masks

The most neutral of the fruits and vegetables are the cucumber and papaya. Watermelon, fig, raw horse-radish, onion, persimmon, sweet green pepper, casaba melon and banana are also quite neutral.

If your skin needs an acid boost because of excess oiliness, these are the most acid foods you can use in a facial: lime, lemon, grape, cranberry, strawberry, pineapple, grapefruit, apple, all in descending order.

Those with dry skin will want less acid foods and they are: cantaloupe, avocado, honeydew melon, olive, lettuce, carrot and parsley. Parsley is also quite effective with oily skin.

You can use any of the foods mentioned as a spontaneous facial, even as you are preparing salads and desserts. Allow the substance to dry on the face just as you would a real facial, and wash it off with tepid water.

For a formal vegetable or fruit facial, peel and mash any of the above foods and add to a binding substance. For excessively oily skin you might want to concentrate on drying substances such as buttermilk, yogurt, clay, earth, egg white. Always add a few *drops* of apple cider vinegar.

For dry skin the banana, honey, sour cream or egg yolk are quite helpful. Add a tablespoon of your favourite oil, and a few *drops* of apple cider vinegar.

Honey is a neutral binder.

Hot-weather Cucumber Mask

ice cube	
peeled cucumber	
honey	½ teaspoon
milk	2 tablespoons
(for additional thickening add ½ teaspoon powdered milk)	
witch hazel	½ teaspoon
peppermint extract	5 drops
or	
peppermint oil	2 drops

Blend and crush ice cube, cucumber, honey, milk, witch hazel and peppermint. Pat mask on face. Dry for 15 minutes or more, wash off with tepid water, pat dry. Close pores with ice cold astringent. (Unless you have a sensitive skin or broken veins on face. In which case you must use only a mild astringent.) This is a refreshing, cooling summer mask.

Tightening Cucumber Mask

peeled cucumber	
cider vinegar or lemon juice	¼ teaspoon
witch hazel	1 teaspoon
ethyl alcohol	1 teaspoon
egg white	1

Extract the juice of cucumber in a juicer or blend 1 small cucumber quickly (otherwise it liquefies too much in the blender) and add either cider vinegar or pure lemon juice, witch hazel, ethyl alcohol.

Take the mixture out of the blender and add 1 whipped egg white. Pat this mixture on the face and allow it to dry for 15 minutes or more. Wipe off with tepid water and a soft flannel. Pat dry. Pat on herbal or favourite astringent.

Two other optional *tightening* products for this or *any* other mask would be ¼ teaspoon of simple tincture of benzoin, or a pinch of alum powder.

Carrot Mask

Carrots are rich in vitamin A, which is very useful in treating all skin problems and allergy attacks. If you have a persistent skin problem you should explore the benefits of eating lots of raw carrots and drinking carrot juice. A fresh carrot-juice cocktail from an extractor-juicer is a quick pick-me-up too. If you are lucky enough to live where you can obtain pesticide-free carrots they will taste quite different from most carrots in the market. They are much sweeter and there is absolutely no taste of chemicals.

To make a carrot-juice or pulp facial add either whipped egg white or honey or buttermilk.

Parsley Facial

Parsley cuts down on the excess oiliness of the skin and adds sheen. It is too harsh to rub into the skin, so you have to extract its elements with boiling water and let it cool for 15 minutes or longer, or juice it in the blender or juice extractor. If you like, you can also use carrot juice or celery juice or apple juice in this vegetable facial. All are helpful to the skin. These same vegetables are helpful internally and should be used daily raw or as juice to help clear the system of impurities. These juices are very thin and therefore difficult to apply. They can be thickened with buttermilk, sour cream, yogurt, honey, egg white or egg yolk or with kaolin or fuller's earth, depending on your skin quality. Cabbage juice is also used occasionally to restore skin, but I find the smell unpleasant.

Ovid's Beautifying Facial

Have you ever wondered how the ladies of antiquity took care of their skin-nourishing problems? Ovid recorded the following ingredients in a recipe, saying: "Every woman who covers her face with this will make it more brilliant than a mirror."

I like this recipe, but Ovid uses such large amounts that an entire girl's school could take a facial at the same time, so I merely list his ingredients.

Ovid advises the following: lentils, eggs—ground into a powder and then a flour and passed through a sieve (try powdered eggs). Add powdered narcissus bulbs (these and several other bulbs mentioned through this book are excellent cosmetic aids), gum benzoin (you could use simple tincture of benzoin), honey and wheat flour.

Gardener's Special Facial

This complexion mask was reported to be effective in producing a bright and pure-looking skin. It will undoubtedly appeal to gardeners, for it relies on equal amounts of the seed of melon, pumpkin, gourd and cucumber. The seeds must be dried and then pounded until they are reduced to a powder. Add enough cream to make this flour into a paste and add enough milk to dilute it. For aroma you might want to add a few drops of lemon oil, or some other aromatic oil. Pat on face. Keep the mask on for 15 minutes or more. Wash off with tepid water. Close pores with astringent.

Other special masks for skin problems, including spots, dry skin, large pores, oily skin, broken (thread) veins, rough skin, or double chin, can be found under the appropriate headings, or by consulting the index.

5. SPOTS

Blackheads, Whiteheads, Pimples, Acne

"Out damned spot!" Most of us have stood in front of a mirror at some time and wished that a "spot" would disappear. No one likes whiteheads, blackheads or pimples, particularly the kind that can lead to acne.

To cure these blemishes you have to know their cause. Your 21 square feet of skin has many important functions. Besides helping you to breathe and exude perspiration (1 quart a day and up to 20 quarts if you are exercising or tense), it also helps to eliminate toxic material through its millions of pores. Which is why you sometimes get pimples when your stomach is upset. Your skin also reflects your feelings—goose flesh when you are cold or scared, and pimples when you are unhappy or tense. Your complexion is a reflection of the total you—how much good sleep you have, the food you are eating or not eating, your feelings, your ability adequately to discharge waste materials and your cleanliness.

But this doesn't explain the trauma of sudden and disastrous attacks of whiteheads, blackheads and pimples when young people reach puberty. At the time you care most about your clean and healthy looks, nature somehow foils you. How? Your body has a natural oil-manufacturing system which exudes sebum— nature's cold cream. Too much sebum and your skin is oily. Too little sebum and your skin is dry.

During adolescence there is a great stirring of both female and male hormone production, and if there is the *slightest* imbalance of these hormones, the sebaceous glands are forced to send up *extra* sebum. That would be all right if you could just wipe off this excess oil. But it comes up through the pores, and if there is some sebum stuck there already, you get a white "bump" which, if not almost immediately removed by either steam facial, gentle friction or an enriching scrub, hardens in 7 or 8 hours. The hardened oil is called a whitehead and becomes a blackhead when oxidized by the air.

Sometimes the excess sebum emerges only *under* the skin and causes a reddish bump which, if not immediately cleared, becomes infected when the body's defence apparatus, the white corpuscles, create those most dreaded of all adolescent scourges —pus-filled pimples. A few of these and you have acne. And if you touch your face a lot, and don't keep it scrupulously clean, or if the pus oozes out, the acne spreads.

Girls are frequently troubled by such pimples a few days before their menstrual period when the female hormone production of oestrogen is low and the male hormone androgen takes over and causes a slight imbalance. But boys are the worst sufferers from this sudden production of sebum, since male puberty brings on an excess production of male hormones.

However, hormones are not the only cause of excess oiliness of the skin; it is also related to the food you eat. All B complex vitamins are known to affect skin and hair. To increase your intake of all Bs take brewer's yeast daily—you will find it quite tasty in the flake form dissolved in a strong fruit juice; and liver three times a week, or liver tablets every day. Yeast regulates the secretions of the skin.

Another really effective acne aid is lecithin, which emulsifies and breaks down fatty globules in the blood. This frequently works wonders. One grown man I know was able to control serious acne on his body with doses of lecithin after failing with every other treatment. The suggested daily dose is 2 tablespoons of the granules dissolved in some fruit juice, or 6 capsules. You can combine the lecithin and the yeast and drink them together.

Herbal drinks and vegetable juices are also very useful in clearing blemishes. Carrot juice can be drunk alone—up to a pint a day—or combined with spinach; use about twice as much carrot juice as you do spinach. Or you can use a combination of carrots, lettuce and spinach, in the proportions 5 ounces of carrots, 2 of lettuce, ½ ounce of spinach. Or increase the spinach to 1 ounce and add ½ ounce of parsley. A simple but amazingly effective treatment is lots and lots of water—8 to 10 glasses a day.

Acne Don'ts

New York dermatologist Irwin Lubowe considers that peanut butter, most nuts, fatty or fried foods, shellfish, iodized salt and animal fats, particularly butter, are bad for young people worried about acne. "Too much iodine in the system stimulates acne, and iodized salt, spices and shellfish all contain iodine," he notes. Also on Dr. Lubowe's NO list are chocolate, cocoa, sticky puddings, pork products, pies and pastries of all kinds, Coca-Cola and other soft drinks, sharp cheeses, dates, sugar, homogenized milk, hot coffee and hot tea or alcohol (these last because they dilate the capillaries of the face).

Other Causes of Acne

Sometimes infections in the system cause acne—so, if you are doing all the right things and your acne is still spreading, check your teeth and your tonsils. For such infections many people find that an increase in the intake of vitamin C is most helpful.

Worry and tension sometimes cause acne. While it is difficult to force yourself to become a more relaxed person in general, one way is to make sure of a good night's sleep. There are many suggestions for the treatment of insomnia in Chapter IX.

Exercise—indoor and outdoor—can dissipate tension. Yoga exercises are being increasingly accepted here in the West as a method of achieving body control, harmony and relaxation. If there are no classes in your area, you can obtain books and records which will help you to learn the various movements, stretches and breathing methods.

Blackhead and Whitehead Cleansers

The best *defence* is *offence*. If you are prone to blackheads and / or whiteheads, try some of these night-cleaning, skin-toning remedies. All of them have been known for generations, and some for many centuries, and were used effectively and happily in the simpler past. Some are preventives, some are preventive-cleansers. All work. You have to experiment and see which one of them suits your temperament and your skin.

Herbal Steam Facial

One of the easiest of all blackhead cleansers is one which my mother learned from her mother and which had been passed down for generations. It is the simple and effective herbal facial (steam) bath.

Boil a pint of water and pour over 2 tablespoons of *any* complexion herb. Suggested herbs are chamomile, yarrow, lady's mantle, nettle, fennel, comfrey, houseleek, lime flowers. Improvise a towel tent-hood and allow the steam to penetrate your face for 10 minutes or more. Your pores should then be wide open and the blackheads can be pushed out by circling them with clean cotton wool or tissue. Do not touch the blackheads with your hands. Close pores with cool water or astringent. If the blackheads are still imbedded in your pores, take a long steamy bath (epsom salt baths are a help) and then try using the herbal steam facial again. The blackheads will probably come out more easily. For more resistant blackheads, try the almond oil facial or the Never-fail Blackhead Remover below.

Almond Oil Facial

Gently pat sweet almond oil over the area of visible blackheads. Apply hot towels on the blackhead area several times. In addition to the bath and the facial this will soften deeply imbedded blackheads, and will help loosen them enough for you to push them out with a tissue or cotton wool.

Never-fail Blackhead Remover

An emergency remover when everything else has failed is the following special facial on the visible blackheads (after you have already opened your pores with a steam facial and bath):

epsom salts	1 tablespoon
iodine (preferably white)	3 drops
boiling water	1 cup
flannels	several

Dissolve epsom salts and iodine into the boiling water, which should be kept hot either on an electric hot tray or in another pan of boiling water. Soak a soft flannel in the hot epsom salts solution and then press on imbedded blackhead area. Keep changing flannels and use them very hot. Press with tissue or handkerchief to remove blackhead or whitehead.

Honey Cleanser

Honey is a splendid blackhead and facial cleanser as well as skin nourisher and healer. Heat about 4 tablespoons of honey and gently pat over blackhead area or entire face. If your face is particularly blemished, add a small amount of natural wheat germ to the honey, which will draw the blemishes to the surface of the skin. Honey-Wheat Germ Mask is antiseptic and toning. Keep on face 15 minutes or more. Relax while you wait. Wash off with clean cloth and tepid water. Close pores with astringent. Honey can also be used with the following cereal scrubs.

Cereal Scrubs

Blackheads can also be expelled with a nourishing oatmeal or almond meal-paste mask. You can cook up some old-fashioned oatmeal as if you were making porridge, following the directions on the packet, then add almond meal and gently plaster your face with this paste. You can use this as a daily scrub, as did many famous beauties of the past.

A modern version of the oatmeal scrub is colloidal oatmeal. This needs no prior preparation. Just add water and use as your non-allergic daily scrub. This is marvellous for people with delicate or allergic skin. There are also oatmeal "soaps" on the market which contain no soap and are excellent for allergic skin or persistent skin rashes.

Another old-fashioned combination which uses *three* blackhead cleansers and preventers is a combination of 3 tablespoons of colloidal oatmeal, a teaspoon of white wine and a teaspoon of lemon. This can be used several times a day. Lemon attracts mould so make it up fresh, or keep the scrub in the refrigerator, in which case you can make up a larger batch.

Yet another blackhead cleanser combines 4 ounces of powdered colloidal oatmeal with 2 ounces of powdered almond meal, ½ ounce of fuller's earth and about an ounce of a liquid herbal soap, or glycerine soap shavings. You can keep this in an attractive container in your bathroom and use it as a liquid scrub by adding water. Rub into the blackhead area to make a lather.

Lemon Cleansers

You will find lemon juice, by itself or combined with other products, an ideal blackhead preventer, as it is antiseptic, and cleansing, and restores acidity to the skin. Use fresh strained lemon juice whenever you can, or mix with equal parts of rose water or orange or elder flower water.

An effective lemon and whipped egg-white preparation was used for centuries for control of blackheads and for complexion care. Juice ½ lemon. Strain. Whip up an egg white. Heat together in a basin or stainless steel pan until they thicken. Place in jar, label, *and keep refrigerated*. To preserve it without refrigeration, simply add 3–4 drops of simple tincture of benzoin.

Milk

Milk is very useful in blackhead prevention. In fact Dr. Anna Kingsford, a very knowledgeable doctor of the late nineteenth century, wrote that "the only way permanently to rid the face of blackheads is to wash with water as warm as possible, and bathe the face (with a sponge) for 10 minutes in *tepid* milk."

A skin-soothing *herbal milk* can be made by soaking 4 tablespoons of yarrow or chamomile in 2 cups of cold milk for several hours. Keep refrigerated and heat slightly before using as wash.

Lanolin Pimple Cleanser-cream

rose water	2 pints
apples	2
celery	2 tablespoons
fennel	2 tablespoons
barley meal	¼ ounce
egg whites	4
anhydrous lanolin	1 teaspoon

Simmer together, in 2 pints of rose water, 2 peeled apples, the celery, fennel and barley meal. Add beaten whites of egg and lanolin. Squeeze the mixture through a strainer. Beat mixture until smooth. Place in labelled jar. Keep in refrigerator.

Camphor Cucumber Pimple Drying Mask

(This can also be used as a circulation boosting mask.)
Camphor BP* contains a soothing and drying ingredient.

camphor BP	¼ cake
egg white	1
peeled cucumber	1
lemon juice	¼ teaspoon
ethyl alcohol	1 teaspoon
witch hazel	1 teaspoon
(or no alcohol, 2 teaspoons witch hazel)	
peppermint oil or extract	3 drops

optional

simple tincture of benzoin	5 drops
or	
powdered alum	¼ teaspoon

* Camphor BP is natural camphor, obtainable from chemists—not mothballs, which are made from a synthetic chemical not to be used on the skin.

Crush camphor, add to whipped egg white and cucumber. Blend together. Add lemon juice (or cider vinegar), alcohol, witch hazel, peppermint oil or extract. Blend again. For extra tightening action add simple tincture of benzoin or powdered alum. Put mask on face. Allow to dry. Remove in 15 or 20 minutes. Wash off with tepid water. Rinse again. Close pores with strong astringent.

Additional Blemish Controllers

Fresh cucumber slices or juice, or crushed watercress leaves or juice, can be patted on the face each night and washed off the next morning. Or use any of the following herbs, patted on the face. Allow to dry. If comfortable, leave on overnight and wash off next morning. If not, wash off after 15 minutes.

Decoction: Either horsetail, oak bark, silverweed, leaves and roots of gladwin (a *fleur de lis* iris) decocted in water. Wormwood decocted in vinegar. Cuckoo-pint leaves decocted in milk. Don't drink the decoction; gladwin and cuckoo-pint are both poisonous plants.

Salve: Rue flowers and myrtle leaves crushed together and added to an ointment or cream.

Powder: Crushed lupin seeds.

Sap: Daisy juice from stalk—in spring. Slit the bark of willow or birch in spring to release sap. In *Delights for Ladies* by Sir Hugh Platt (1600), I found the following under the charming heading, "A Secret Not Known To Many":

To Take Away Spots and Freckles From the Face and Hands
The sappe that issueth of a Birch tree in great abundance, being opened in March or April, with a receiver of glasse set under the boring thereof to receive the same, doth perform the same most excellently and maketh the skin very cleare.

Infusion: Pimpernel, patience, alone or combined. Red clover.

Compound: Touch each acne pimple with compound spirit of horse-radish.

Internal Blemish Controls

The following will flush the system of impurities: infusion of wild pansy; pellitory of the wall with distilled water and a small amount of sugar; and a decoction of boiled roots of quick (or couch) grass, silver mantle, beard of Indian corn, and restharrow. Drink several times a day to clear eruptions. These drinks will increase the flow of urine.

Freckles

There are two kinds of freckles—sun freckles, which come and go, and chronic or "cold" freckles. If you don't care for them you can bleach the freckles with various foods and herbs.

Bleaches

All herbal and food bleaches tend to be drying for the skin. To make sure your face and hands don't get too dry from these treatments, oil the freckles area afterwards, unless you already have an oily skin and want to cure it.

Pat any of the following "lotions" on the face or hands and allow to dry from 15 minutes to several hours. Wash off with tepid water. Pat dry again. Close pores with gentle astringent. Pat on oil or nourishing cream.

Buttermilk is a gentle bleach.

Equal parts of lemon juice mixed with either elder flower or rose water.

Two tablespoons of grated fresh horse-radish in cider vinegar and made into a paste.

Two tablespoons of grated fresh horse-radish simmered in milk. Make up into a paste.

Fruits and vegetables with high vitamin C content can also be used to bleach freckles. Make a paste mask of rose-hip powder and small additions of the juice of either parsley, potato, lemon, strawberry or cucumber. Pat on face. Allow to dry. Remove with warm water after 15 minutes. Oil face and use nourishing cream afterwards.

Bleaching herbs which can be used in facials or in infused complexion water are: lime flowers, elder flowers, lady's mantle and chickweed. Any lactic acid product added to elder flower distilled water or elder flower infusion will increase the whitening action of the elder flower. Pat on face. Allow to dry. Wash off with tepid water 15 minutes later. Use cream afterwards.

Brown Spots

Liver spots, or age spots, are attributed to a lack of certain vitamins, in particular vitamin E. Other nutritionists mention the need for additional vitamin C in the diet since this vitamin is depleted as one gets older, and also the need for additional vitamin B, particularly B_2 and riboflavin. But it is unwise to dose yourself with only one B vitamin unless your doctor says that you have a deficiency, as this sometimes causes another imbalance. It is better to eat a tablespoon of brewer's yeast which is high in *all* the B vitamins, or use a high level balanced B vitamin. The Bs help with all skin dryness, redness and irritations.

Any of the herbs that help eliminate freckles can also be used as external aids for liver spots. Dr. Jarvis in *Folk Medicine* recommends the application of castor oil until the spots disappear.

Moles

Moles are raised brown bumps. They are similar to freckles, both being due to uneven pigmentation. It is said that everyone has at least one little mole. A folk remedy to reduce moles is equal parts of castor oil and fresh cranberry juice.

6. OILY SKIN

Oily skin may be hard to control, but it does have the virtue of keeping wrinkles away for a long, long time. Oiliness comes from excess sebum when a slight imbalance within the system forces the sebaceous glands to send up more oil than is needed.

There are many ways of controlling an oily skin: from *within* by changing food habits to exclude rich and fried foods, and to include more greens and certain herbs; and from *without* by daily herbal steaming, deep pore scrubbing with herbs and grease-cutting foods which absorb dirt and grease, and with herbal and food astringents which degrease the face and body and close the pores after cleansing. The best internal emulsifier is lecithin, a by-product of soy beans. Take 2 tablespoons of lecithin granules daily.

Since many adolescents have an oily skin and consequently have trouble with blackheads, whiteheads and pimples, as well as acne, I have included a more complete discussion of this problem in Section 5 of this chapter.

Herbal Steam Facial

Steaming is very good for an oily skin as it cuts the external grease and deep-cleans the clogged pores, and allows you to push out the blackheads and whiteheads easily, and therefore to avoid pimples.

A description of the steam facial can be found in Section 2.

Cleaners

Fuller's earth can be used to absorb excess oil on the face. Better still are any number of absorbent cereals, which can be used as daily scrubs for the face and body. These include bran, oatmeal, almond meal and cornmeal. Colloidal oatmeal (suspended and ready to use as it is) makes a marvellous, non-allergenic scrub which will leave your skin velvety smooth.

Helpers

Lemon juice and water, cider vinegar and water are splendid cleansing and after-cleansing substances, and they will help restore the acid covering which your skin needs for protection. Tepid milk is an excellent healing substance for daily cleansing and blackhead prevention. White wine is a wonderful after-cleansing, degreasing substance. Buttermilk, beaten egg white and yogurt all help to control excessively oily skin, and can be used directly on the face or in combination with astringent herbs.

Yarrow, chamomile, lady's mantle, elder flower, sage can all help cut down on excess lubrication of the skin. They are all astringent. Many herbalists recommend drinking a cup of yarrow tea every day to cut down on skin oiliness. To make a strong infusion, use 2 tablespoons of yarrow to a glass and a half of boiling water. Steep and strain. Drink warm or cold. Of particular interest also is horsetail, which is one of the oldest plants on earth, and is quite stimulating to the skin. For a horsetail wash, use a decoction. Use infusion for the other herbs.

Oily Skin Masks

Cucumber, parsley and cabbage are all excellent in controlling oily skin, but cucumber is the easiest to use. Two other foods which are reliable are tomato and buttermilk, both of which can be used in connection with other ingredients in a facial. Yogurt can also be used as a mask-binder and combined with these foods or the herb infusion we have mentioned before. See Sections 4, 7 and 13.

Tomato-lemon

This is a real winner for oily skins, as it combines two astringent skin-nourishing foods. Blend them together in a blender, *or* steep the tomato juice or pulp in the inside of a lemon. After steeping, scrape off the lemon-tomato pulp and splash on your face.

If you haven't time for a whole mask and you tend to have an oily skin, rub the pulp of a tomato or lemon on your face, and wash off with tepid water.

Brewer's Yeast Facial

This facial is very successful for those with oily skins and can be used as a tingling, vitamin-rich, nourishing stimulator twice a week. Stir the yeast powder or flakes into a stiff paste with milk, buttermilk, yogurt, rose water, witch hazel, fuller's earth or kaolin, and pat on to a clean face. Wash off with tepid water and close the pores with strong cold astringent.

Marie Antoinette's Oily Skin Mask

It is interesting to discover that Marie Antoinette was worried about her too oily skin, but she evidently helped keep it under control with this nightly facial:

milk	½ pint
lemon juice	¼ ounce
brandy	½ ounce

Simmer over a gentle flame. Apply to face. Allow to dry. Wash off 15 minutes later with warm water. Rinse with slightly cooler water. Close pores with astringent.

The Duchess of Alba Facial is also good for oily skin; see page 36.

Astringents

There is a complete listing of herb and food astringent substances in Section 13.

7. LARGE PORES

Although large pores are frequently identified with excess sebum, even people with dry skin can have large pore areas on their face. You can keep the problem under control with steam and herbal facials which will keep the area clean, and a large number of foods and herbs which can temporarily tighten the pores.

Any one of the following can be used alone or in combination with each other: beaten egg white, buttermilk, tomato, cornmeal, oatmeal, bran, almond meal, lemon, vinegar and water, alum powder, milk, honey, camphor BP, or the herbs horsetail, sage or yarrow. If you find the substances too watery, add a facial pack thickener like fuller's earth. Your face should be clean and dry before applying the mask. Allow the nourishing herb or food to dry on the face for 20 minutes. Afterwards wash off with tepid water and soft cloth. Pat dry. Close pores with astringent. Herbal and other astringents will be found in Section 13.

If you have a dry skin be sure to use these facials and washes only on the large pore area of your face.

Egg-white Masks

Frothy egg white is one of nature's most successful skin tighteners and drying agents, and is therefore most useful for large pore control. Egg white can be used alone, or in combination with lemon juice or yarrow infusion, or both.

A *tingling* egg-white and cucumber mask is quite simple to make:

peeled cucumber	1
egg white	2
lemon juice	1 teaspoon
ethyl rubbing alcohol 50% (buy best brand)	2 tablespoons
ice cube	
peppermint extract	¼ teaspoon

Peel a cucumber. Whip up egg whites in a blender, then blend together for a few seconds the cucumber, the egg whites, lemon juice, ethyl rubbing alcohol, ice cube and peppermint extract.

The peppermint will create a menthol effect. Keep leftovers in refrigerator in a labelled container and use the next day. For additional tightening effect, add a pinch of alum to the above recipe. Alum is available in powder form at the chemist's.

Another splendid skin tightener is gum arabic, which is available at some chemists. This gum dissolves in double its weight of water, especially heated water. Use 1 teaspoon in 1 ounce of water. Use with egg white alone or with cucumber mask.

Tomato Mask

Tomatoes have a lot of vitamin C and potassium, and are very successful in controlling large pores. You can try squishing a tomato on your face, or use buttermilk, or yogurt, or fuller's earth added to the pulp to make a facial paste. Apply to clean face, allow to dry for 15 minutes. Wash off with tepid water.

Buttermilk Washes

Use as a 15-minute facial and rinse off carefully. Or buttermilk and salt can be blended together to make a paste.

Herb Helpers

All kinds of herbs are helpful in controlling large pores, and possibly camphor BP is the most successful since camphor is soothing and healing as well as tightening. This is of course natural camphor, *not* the "camphor" used in moth prevention— nowadays a synthetic chemical not to be used on the skin. You can buy camphor ice at the chemists, or buy spirits of camphor and use a few drops in rose water or elder flower water as a nightly astringent after you have cleaned your face. You can make a delightful camphor *facial* with a tablespoon of honey, a tablespoon of brandy and 3 drops of spirits of camphor.

In addition, yarrow, horsetail or sage are helpful for large pores, both as facials and taken internally. For a facial, make a strong infusion by adding a cup of boiling water to 2 tablespoons of any of the herbs. Steep for at least 15 minutes. Strain. These can all be used externally with milk, honey, lemon, cider vinegar or *any* of the products mentioned in this section. As stated before, alum powder can be added to any herb for additional skin-tightening power.

Almond Meal

Almonds have a healing, soothing and nourishing effect on the skin and were used in ancient Greece for facials and hand creams. You can use either prepared almond meal and rose water or elder flower water, or you can pulverize your own almonds and make them into a paste with the addition of milk, buttermilk or yogurt. You can also add a few drops of simple tincture of benzoin for its astringent and cleansing qualities, and a pinch of skin-tightening alum powder.

Cornmeal / Oatmeal Mask

These meals are deep pore cleansers. They are extremely nourishing and give the skin a silky texture. Make a thick paste of either cornmeal or oatmeal. Use warm. For a large pore mask you can also add one of the many nourishing liquids such as buttermilk, tomato pulp, cucumber juice, egg white or yarrow, sage or horsetail herb infusion.

Large Pore Astringent

This will help correct coarse large pores, oily or flabby skin:

cucumber juice	1½ ounces
cologne	1 ounce
elder flower water	5 ounces
simple tincture of benzoin	½ ounce

Mix the cucumber juice, cologne and elder flower water and place in an 8-ounce bottle. Add simple tincture of benzoin. Shake slightly.

8. DRY SKIN

Basically it is the excess production of sebum, the skin oil, which causes acne, so those with dry skins are spared the agony and problems of acne pimples. But later on, as the years advance, this plus turns into a minus, for the lack of lubrication from within the body may lead to early wrinkles. Therefore the time to treat dry skin is NOW, and fortunately you can plan an inner and outer programme which will have almost immediate results.

Nutritional Aids

A properly restructured nutritional programme frequently shows results in less than 2 weeks' time. However, don't expect a complete cure so soon, for it will require patience. It won't be enough to cream and moisturize your face from without. You must at the same time make an effort to include high vitamin A, B complex, C and E rich foods in your diet. If your skin is exceptionally dry, or if you are over 40, also add these vitamins to your diet in the form of supplements, remembering that supplements are just what they say they are—and not *substitutes* for nourishing food.

People on fat-free diets often discover that as they lose weight the facial skin begins to sag. Actually, many nutritionists suggest that a completely fat-free diet is a mistake, and it is necessary and advisable to *add* a moderate amount of polyunsaturated oils like safflower, sunflower and sesame to the diet. Incidentally, the fat soluble vitamins A, B and E are not assimilated without fat, and your body cannot manufacture the B vitamins in your intestines without some fat.

Dry-skin Facial Materials

Many foods are moisturizing as well as nourishing and penetrating. For dry skin care, use the following substances alone or in combination with other suggested materials:

The oil of avocado, wheat germ, almond and linseed and grocery store oils like the polyunsaturated safflower, olive and peanut oils are helpful in dry skin care. Lanolin is also very helpful, as are egg *yolk*, apple juice, peach juice, sour cream, honeydrew melon juice, brewer's yeast (internal as well as external), milk, honey, oatmeal, almond meal, crushed almonds, liquid lecithin.

Brewer's Yeast Plan

Brewer's yeast can be helpful to people with either dry or oily skin, since it helps control skin secretions. It is a source of all the B vitamins. Since some skin deficiencies are due to a lack of this vitamin in the diet, a 3-month "assault plan" would include drinking a tablespoon of this yeast in some strong juice such as apple, grape or cranberry each day, and applying a once-a-week facial mask. The brewer's yeast mask sometimes brings out impurities from the system in the form of blotches, although these disappear in a short time. For this reason it is not advisable to use this facial mask just before going out to a party. The mask is made in the following way:

hot water	few drops
honey	1 teaspoon
brewer's yeast	1 tablespoon
milk	1 teaspoon
(or favourite skin oil)	
oil for face	1 teaspoon

Add a few drops of hot water to honey to liquefy it. Blend in dried brewer's yeast. Add either milk or oil to soften. Stir into thick paste. Apply oil base to face. Pat paste on face. Allow to dry for 15 to 30 minutes. Remove with cotton wool or flannel soaked in tepid water. Use a mild astringent such as cucumber, chamomile or witch hazel (see Section 13).

Peach Facial

Use a blended peach plus any of the above materials and/or vitamins A and D for a fine dry skin moisturizing facial treatment.

Oatmeal Facial

Super-fatted colloidal oatmeal makes a very fine nourishing and bleaching facial base. You can add a tablespoon of oatmeal to a tablespoon of almond meal. Add rose water, nettle water, elder flower water or milk. Work this up into a thick paste and gently pat on the neck and face. Allow to dry for at least 15 minutes. Wash off with tepid water. The oatmeal creates a silken effect on the skin.

Vitamin-lanolin Treatment

This is listed in Section 3. It is an excellent treatment and can be used daily.

Cosmetic Vinegar

Vinegar softens dry body skin and is magical with mottled dry body or leg skin. It can be used in the bath as often as needed. Read the directions in Section 14.

Exceptionally Flaky Skin

Use the lemon-water-oil spring cleaner facial listed in Section 4.

Ashy Skin

Many dark or black-skinned people have a winter skin problem when their drying skin turns ashy. Many black-skinned people use Vaseline or mineral oil on the skin for this problem, but neither of these products is suitable for the face, and neither should *ever* be used. Instead, treat the problem as an extreme dry-skin problem. Change the diet and add vitamins as suggested in the beginning of this section, add oils to your salads, and use nourishers and moisturizers frequently on the skin.

Humidifiers

Unfortunately most flats and houses are overheated in the winter time. If you cannot regulate the heat yourself, invest in a home humidifier which releases water back into the air. This will help your family to keep healthier too, as excessive drying of the air dries the membranes of the nose and creates a climate for infection. If you cannot buy a humidifier, keep the windows wide open when you sleep. Or use an atomizer filled with distilled water and a teaspoon of glycerine. Use this in your nose, on your face and in the air whenever possible.

9. ROUGH SKIN

Rough Elbows

Many women neglect this area of the body and accumulate dark, ridged, sandpaper-texture elbows. It is very easy to "cure" this condition. Lemon pulp and peel have a remarkable whitening and softening effect on skin, and you can keep lemon halves on the kitchen sink next to the soap. Give yourself a lemon swabbing every chance you get.

Oatmeal Washes

Leftover breakfast oatmeal can be used as a wash or skin paste on any roughened area. Better still is colloidal oatmeal which needs no preparation. Keep some in a little jar in the bathroom and merely add water to make into hand, face, elbow or body paste and wash. Oatmeal is wonderful for delicate and allergic skin.

Almond Meal Paste

Rough and blotchy skin responds to the healing qualities of almonds. Use either pulverized almonds and milk, or almond meal and milk, or almond oil and honey. Pat on hands and elbows or rough spots. Allow to dry. Rinse off with tepid water. Pat dry. Try adding a pulverized apple to the almonds for increased therapeutic effect.

Cider Vinegar

Cider vinegar plus water in a 1-to-8 proportion will restore the acid covering your skin craves and help keep elbows and other skin areas supple and un-flaky.

White Brandy Chap Chaser

Mix 2 parts of white brandy with 1 part of rose water for a morning and night wash. The brandy gently cleanses the surface of the skin while the rose water counteracts the drying nature of the brandy and leaves the skin natural, soft and flexible.

Narcissus-cucumber-brandy Wash

Another old and respected chap chaser is powdered cucumber roots and narcissus roots soaked in white brandy. Measure a tablespoon to a pint. Use as a morning or night wash.

Daisy Heads Wash

An infusion of daisy heads left on the face to dry is a folk remedy to prevent blotching.

Milk

Warmed milk can cure roughened skin. It can be added to almonds, oatmeal, powdered cucumber roots, powdered narcissus roots or daisy heads.

Milk Lotion

milk	½ pint
glycerine	½ ounce
bicarbonate of soda	½ ounce
borax	½ ounce

Warm the milk and slowly add glycerine, bicarbonate of soda and borax until all three dissolve. Place in labelled bottle in refrigerator. This is an excellent lotion for roughened skin.

Rose Water and Glycerine

You can buy this very healing substance in any chemist's. For a recipe see Chapter VII.

Herb Chap Chasers

Comfrey is a remarkable skin-healing herb which strengthens cell formation and helps cure rough or chapped areas. It is high in mucilage, as is also the common mallow, from which the confection marshmallow was originally made. Marigold flowers are also good healers. Make an infusion of comfrey or marigold, or a decoction of mallow root. Add to any hand ointment or cream, to rose water and glycerine combined or various washes mentioned previously.

Eczema

Eczema is an extremely irritating and tenacious skin problem, and I have chosen to list it under rough skin because almost nothing is rougher. According to nutritional experts, this condition can be cleared up if the body takes in an adequate diet rich in linoleic acid and all B vitamins. They write of a man whose body was covered with weeping sores of moist eczema (there is also a dry kind), who was cured by taking a heaped tablespoon of yeast with each meal and between meals for 2 weeks.

For dry, scaly skin eczema, Adelle Davis recommends 1 to 3 tablespoons of safflower oil or other cold pressed oils as part of the daily diet. Many allergic people find eczema appears quite suddenly when they are under stress. This can usually be cleared up with a diet heavy in B_{12} foods and liver and other anti-stress foods.

A folk cure for eczema is eating huge amounts of watercress; another is eating one raw potato a day. An infusion wash of wormwood is recommended by Father Kunzle in the case of scabs, eczema and other eruptions of the face. Nelson Coon notes that 9-grain cress tablets are prescribed by homeopaths and osteopaths for eczema.

10. THREAD VEINS

Small thread veins or broken veins on the face can respond to careful treatment and increase in vitamin C and rutin products. Rutin can be obtained from buckwheat products or tablets, while vitamin C intake can be increased with either a high-grade *natural* supplement or such foods as parsley, grapefruit, oranges or rose hips. *Don't* drink coffee, tea or alcohol since these dilate the veins. Instead use herb teas, peppermint, chamomile and particularly coltsfoot, which is soothing internally and externally. And never use steam saunas, or facial steaming, or any hot water on the skin, only tepid water.

Coltsfoot Compresses

Coltsfoot can be used externally as well as internally as a tea. Before applying, clean your face with a mild cleanser. Pat some warm milk on your face, especially in the thread vein area.

Allow to dry for 15 minutes. Wash off with soft cloth and tepid water. To make the compress, make a milk or water infusion with coltsfoot following the directions in Chapter I. Place the warm steeped herb in a cloth napkin. Apply to the veined area just after it has been washed free of the warm milk.

Yeast / Wheat Germ Mask

This mask is nourishing for the skin, and weekly applications for several months will alleviate the vein condition.

whole egg	1 teaspoon
dried brewer's yeast	1 teaspoon
wheat germ	1 teaspoon
wheat germ oil	1 teaspoon

Blend together egg, yeast, wheat germ, wheat germ oil. Gently pat on face. Allow to dry for 15 minutes. Wash the facial off with soft cloth and tepid water. Pat face dry again. Apply a gentle coating of wheat germ oil, or any other skin nourishing oil.

Dry Skin

Many people with thread veins on their face have dry skin areas which need special attention. A mask of brewer's yeast and wheat germ, followed by wheat germ oiling of the area, should help with this condition. Another effective food combination is a green pepper and honey mask. Liquidize half a small pepper and add a tablespoon of honey. After the face is thoroughly cleansed, dab it with the inner rind of orange, lemon or grapefruit. Then add the mask. For other remedies for dry skin, see Section 8.

Oily Skin

The herbs and foods suggested in Section 6 will help to control the excessive secretion of oil to the skin. The following mask should also help.

Make a mixture of parsley juice and honey and pat over the face. For particularly oily skin add also several drops of either lemon juice or cider vinegar to the mask. Dry on face for 15 minutes. Remove later with tepid water.

Marigold Lotion

Gardeners will be delighted to discover an additional use for this pungent flower which is so healing to the skin. Steep the leaves in boiling water and leave for 20 minutes to 3 hours. Strain and pat on face. This is a very old folk remedy for the thread-vein condition.

11. DOUBLE CHIN

The chin, neck and jawline are often the first areas to sag. This reflects several negative conditions which you can gradually overcome or prevent—lack of consistent circulation and exercise for that area, lack of protein, need for more salads and raw vegetables and need for increased vitamin E, both internally and externally. This vitamin is seriously depleted in women approaching their menopause.

According to Dr. Maximilian Le Witter, a physician also concerned with vitamins and food, vitamin E is one of the most remarkable of the vitamins, but one should be careful with the dosage of supplements, since intake is tied in with blood pressure. However, this vitamin is widely distributed in plants and animal tissue. Particularly rich sources are green leaves, and oil from cereal seeds, especially wheat germ oil, and the vegetable oils soy bean, corn, cottonseed and peanut in that order. Dairy products like milk, butter, eggs have vitamin E, as do liver, various fruits and brown rice, barley, rye, nuts, legumes. You can easily increase your daily intake of vitamin E through a diet which also includes apples, sweet corn and dried beans.

After increasing your daily intake of both protein and vitamin E there are several daily exercises you should try.

Neck Exercises

My favourite neck exercise is the clockwise and counter-clockwise *circular* motion. Do each 3 times. Try to make the motions fluid. You will find this extremely relaxing. Inhale deeply and hold breath until you return to first position.

Move the neck forward and back—the *"yes, yes"* motion. Inhale with head upright. Forward—hold—exhale. Lift up. Inhale; three times.

Move the neck from side to side—the *"no, no"* motion. Inhale deeply with head upright. Exhale with each slow side motion. Repeat 3 times.

Head push. With elbows resting on table, clasp hands at the back of the neck on the lower part of the head. Inhale. Gently press head down to chest. Exhale. Return to forward, front position. Inhale. Press head gently to right shoulder. Exhale. Return to forward position. Inhale. Press head to left shoulder. Exhale. Return. Inhale. Press head back. Exhale. Return upright. Inhale.

Double chin push. This isometric exercise will prevent a double chin, but it is an extremely difficult exercise to perfect.

With elbows resting on table, mesh fingers of both hands together in a "Here's the church" clasp and push against your chin. At the same time push your chin against your locked hands. Push equally hard on chin and hands and hold pressure for a count of 20. (You might prefer starting with a count of 5 and working up to a count of 20.) You should be very tired from the exercise.

Once you have mastered the exercises, added the foods rich in vitamin E and perhaps added a small amount of vitamin E supplement to your diet, you should experiment with the following nourishing neck massages.

Oil Treatments

There are any number of rich oils which can nourish your sensitive and dry neck area. The easiest of all would be a nightly rub of wheat germ oil massaged *upwards* from the bottom of the neck to the chin. Some people love the smell of wheat germ oil. If it doesn't appeal to you, use slightly warmed peanut or corn oil. Cocoa butter would be helpful in nightly massage, and even better than plain cocoa butter is a double boiler version with lanolin.

Cocoa Butter Neck Smoother

cocoa butter	1 tablespoon
lanolin	1 tablespoon
wheat germ oil	½ cup
(or corn or peanut oil)	

optional

water	4 tablespoons

Melt all 3 oils in the top of a double boiler until all are completely dissolved. Adding water makes it easier to spread. Place in a labelled jar. Refrigerate. Shake before using. Cloudiness does not impair the mixture.

Brewer's Yeast Facial

brewer's yeast	1 tablespoon
wheat germ oil	1 tablespoon
egg yolk	1

Blend together. Apply gently (do not rub) over clean neck and face area. Allow to dry 15 to 20 minutes. Wash off with tepid water. Use soft flannel or absorbent cotton wool.

Hollywood Double Chin Treatment

glycerine	1 teaspoon
epsom salts	½ teaspoon
simple tincture of benzoin	
(or peppermint extract)	5 drops
absorbent cotton wool	5-inch pad
elastic bandage	enough to go round head and chin

Mix glycerine, epsom salts and benzoin or peppermint together. Place on pad of cotton wool. Place under chin. Tie on the elastic bandage. Use several times a week, perhaps while doing chores or watching TV.

12. SUNBATHING

Should one indulge in sunbathing or not? Mild suntan from sports or outdoor work can't be helped, but excessive sun-worshipping has now been found to be destructive. You should avoid long hours in the sun, because it dries the skin and pre-disposes it not only to future ridges, flakiness and wrinkles, but also to skin cancer. Another problem is depletion of your internal vitamin B, for these vitamins have to help your body to form the tanning colour, melanin. Also, if your body happens to be deficient in vitamin C, you may get a blotchy tan, which you sometimes see on people at the beach and pool. Anaemic people frequently cannot tan well because they lack some of the B vitamins, and the mineral copper. The moral is that, if you are obliged or like to be in the sun a lot, be sure to eat plenty of the vitamin C rich foods like citrus fruits, rose hips, cantaloupe, strawberries, tomatoes and a great many vitamin B foods such as eggs, liver, lean meat, poultry, wheat germ, yeast and un-refined cereals. An excellent all-round B complex food supplement is dried brewer's yeast, which can be added to food or to fruit juice.

Susceptibility to Sunburn

Adelle Davis writes that people susceptible to sunburn have been able to tolerate more exposure when taking 1,000 milligrams daily of the B vitamin PABA (para-aminobenzoic acid), and that using PABA as an ointment has allowed even delicate skinned redheads to surf and sunbathe. PABA is available in most ordinary chemists.

Tanning Lotions

Sesame is one of the polyunsaturated nut oils which penetrates and softens the skin, and it is the one which most fully absorbs the ultra-violet rays of the sun. It is therefore a wonderful natural tanning aid.

If you are going swimming you might decide to use the oil only, since it resists water, but the following is a better tanning lotion:

anhydrous lanolin	¼ cup
sesame oil	¼ cup
water	¾ cup

Melt lanolin in top of double boiler. Blend together immediately with sesame oil and water. Pour in labelled jar. Refrigerate.

If you possess a nut grinder, try grinding a handful of *sesame seeds* to make seed lotion. Blend it with a drop of water. Keep in refrigerator or add a preservative such as ¼ teaspoon of ethyl alcohol or witch hazel.

Cucumbers are also a time-honoured protection against the sun.

cucumber	1 small
glycerine	½ teaspoon
rose water	½ teaspoon

Peel and chop cucumber. Squeeze out juice. Mix with glycerine and rose water.

Sunburn Aids

To be used externally:

The mashed pulp of cucumber.
Raw grated potato or potato juice.
Nettle or sage tea.
Strong solution of any ordinary tea. The tannic acid and theobromine in tea help remove heat from the sunburn.
Beaten egg white, combined with 1 teaspoon of honey and ½ teaspoon of witch hazel.
A tablespoon each of witch hazel, olive oil and glycerine combined.
Diluted solution of vinegar and water.
Equal parts of vinegar and olive oil.

Skin Whiteners—Sunburn Bleaches

You can revitalize and whiten the skin with ordinary buttermilk or yogurt, lemon and egg white, milk and lemon, potatoes, ivy twigs, grapes and several flower waters. Remember, though, that all these are drying agents and are best used by those with oily complexions.

A herb mask can be made by infusing cowslip, lily of the valley, fennel or elder flower in boiling water and steeping for an hour. Strain. Add a tablespoon of either buttermilk or yogurt for a bleaching mask.

Pomade de Seville

egg white
lemon juice   equal amounts

Beat egg and lemon together. Set over slow fire. Stir until mixture thickens. Label jar and keep in refrigerator. This is a popular Spanish sunburn bleach which I learnt from the wife of a bull ranch owner.

Mild Bleach

lemon	1 slice
milk	½ cup

Soak lemon in milk. Strain. Pat on face and leave overnight.

Lemon Cream

sweet cream	2 teaspoons
milk	½ pint
lemon	1
brandy	3 ounces
alum powder	pinch
sugar	1 teaspoon

Combine cream and milk. Add lemon juice, brandy, alum and sugar. Simmer for 3 minutes. Skin. When cool place in labelled jar and use. Refrigerate.

Grape Lotion

Grapes are acid, but make a milder face bleach than lemon. This recipe also works, though less well, with ripe green grapes.

unripe green grapes	1 bunch
powdered alum	1 tablespoon
salt	1 teaspoon

Moisten grapes in water. Sprinkle with a mixture of powdered alum and salt. Wrap grapes in brown paper. Bake in hot ashes or slow oven for 15 minutes. Squeeze juice of grapes and wash face with the liquid. Allow to dry for 15 minutes. Wash off with tepid water. This is a very old recipe which is claimed to remove freckles, tan and/or sunburn.

13. ASTRINGENTS

Astringents are tonic and bracing for the skin. They are pore closers and can be used for cutting down excess skin oiliness, particularly after using a cleansing cream. They are also very helpful after shaving.

Bear in mind that all astringents contract the skin slightly, if only for a while, and are also somewhat drying.

Cucumber

As far back as the fifteenth century there are mentions of cooling, pore closing, cleansing properties of this everyday vegetable. There is a hormone in cucumber, by the way, which makes it an anti-wrinkle aid. Moreover its pH is 5.48, while that of the skin is 5.5. The cucumber can be peeled and simply lathered on the face even after a facial steam bath, or before the steam bath as a light cleanser.

Even better than the plain cucumber is the cooling, satiny, mashed or grated peeled cucumber plus ¼ teaspoon of honey, blended or mixed. Bottle, label and refrigerate, since no home cucumber product lasts very long.

For an infallible toner mix three important astringents, cucumber, witch hazel, and egg white, *all of which can be used alone*. The combination of the three together creates a delightful feeling of smoothness and skin vitality:

peeled cucumber	
witch hazel	1 teaspoon
rose water	1 teaspoon
egg white	

optional

honey	¼ teaspoon
yogurt	¼ teaspoon

Mash a whole peeled cucumber. Add witch hazel, rose water, and beaten, frothy egg white. Blend or mix with an electric mixer. Place in labelled jar in the refrigerator. The honey, while not essential, is antiseptic and helps to nourish and cleanse the skin. The yogurt is also cleansing and adds a bleaching action.

Other cucumber masks will be found in Section 4. There is a camphor-cucumber circulation and anti-pimple mask in Section 5.

Egg White

Egg white alone, or added to other ingredients, is very astringent and drying. To use, first cleanse your face, then pat on a frothy, beaten egg white. Allow to dry for 5 to 15 minutes. Wash off with tepid water.

Witch Hazel

The American Indians used poultices of witch hazel twig and bark to bring down the swellings from wounds. It is also antiseptic and can be used as a pore closer, and for quickly reducing any kind of eye, face or body puffiness. I like to use it ice cold. Many men use it as an after-shave lotion.

Witch Hazel Frappé

honey	1 teaspoon
rose water	¾ cup
witch hazel extract	¼ cup
cider vinegar	½ teaspoon
glycerine	½ teaspoon
spirits of camphor (BP)	½ teaspoon
extract of mint	teaspoon (or 5–10 drops of peppermint oil)
either:	
simple tincture of benzoin	5 drops
or:	
alum	pinch
few drops of green vegetable colouring	

Add honey to rose water and mix thoroughly. Blend in witch hazel, cider vinegar, glycerine, spirits of camphor, extract of mint, tincture of benzoin or pinch of alum. Add green colouring. This preparation will be cloudy-looking, but is a marvellous astringent for every day and for winter-weary skin. Keep away from the eyes. Men can use it as an after-shave bracer.

Strawberry

You can squash strawberries over the face as a bracing, toning astringent which will reduce oiliness and help circulation.

Lady Hamilton's Strawberry Astringent Lotion

brandy	½ pint
strawberries	enough for the brandy to cover
camphor (BP)	½ ounce cake

Find a pretty pint bottle and pour in brandy and as many strawberries as the brandy will cover. Make a cover—a piece of porous bladder rubber from a chemistry set is ideal—and leave in the sun or in a warm place for a week. Saving the brandy, strain the strawberries through cheesecloth or a fine-mesh strainer and reserve them for a special dessert that night, and add fresh strawberries to the brandy until it covers them. Add crumbled camphor and let stand. (This of course is not moth balls, but camphor BP, and is a healing, soothing tonic for the skin.) Strain the second batch of strawberries—but don't eat them this time. Use lotion nightly. The lotion will last indefinitely.

Herb Astringents

There are innumerable herbs with astringent qualities, and among them chamomile is my favourite, especially since it has such remarkable antiseptic qualities. One ancient herbalist claims that, for this purpose, it is 120 times stronger than sea water.

The same chamomile that is used in your herb facial sauna, or ice cold on pads for your eyes, can be used (strained of course) and preferably chilled, as a daily astringent. If your face is especially oily, you might want to make up an infusion of yarrow and chamomile combined or lady's mantle and chamomile. Strain off the herbs, bottle and keep in the refrigerator and use as your astringent-tonic after you clean your face each day. Herbs in such as infusion will last many days outside a refrigerator, but will keep indefinitely under cold conditions.

Sage is another easily obtained astringent herb. It is also cooling to the skin. Nettle is a cleansing, purifying herb, as well as being astringent, styptic and stimulating.

Bayberry bark and white oak bark are also mildly astringent, while bistort root is the strongest herb astringent known.

Long-lasting Herbal Astringent

herb extract	1 ounce
glycerine	1 teaspoon
simple tincture of benzoin	¼ teaspoon
boric acid powder	¼ teaspoon
witch hazel	3 tablespoons

optional

peppermint extract	½ teaspoon

First make a herbal extract (with alcohol; See chapter I). Add glycerine, simple tincture of benzoin and boric acid powder which has previously been dissolved in the witch hazel. Add peppermint extract for extra tightening and tingling effect.

14. COSMETIC VINEGARS

Hardly anyone thinks of vinegar as almost the perfect toiletry item. It certainly doesn't evoke the same nostalgia or sense of promise as herbal remedies. Yet it is a complement to all cosmetic herb care. It has been used for thousands of years for hair and skin care, and in folk medicine.

At home we use vinegar for body toning to eliminate fatigue, for hair rinses and light complexion washes. We always use *cider vinegar,* as the malic acid from the apples is good for both the outside and the inside of the human body; cider vinegar restores the acid mantle of the skin, and it can also be combined with honey and boiling water for a drink which I have found works for many different complaints. We buy cider vinegar six bottles at a time—some goes to the bathroom for use in the bath, some goes to concoct creams, lotions and herbal ointments and to be transformed into aromatic or cosmetic vinegar, and some goes into the kitchen, since none of us would start the day without our energy-giving cider vinegar and honey drink.

This preoccupation with vinegar may surprise you; I'm still rather surprised at it myself. But over the years we have learnt how efficient this inexpensive grocery item can be. Vinegar softens the skin and absolutely cancels any itching from dryness. A friend who knew of my interest in ancient remedies wondered if I could recommend something for her husband who suffered from itching on his body, head and face. I suggested a cup of cider vinegar in his bath water. Two days later she telephoned and said her husband felt marvellous and his skin had a completely new texture, and—blessed relief!—didn't feel itchy any more.

The same formula works on dry winter skin—you know, the kind that looks like flaky marble—and skin that's been overdried in the sun. Vinegar should also be added to all hair rinses, or home protein treatments, and it helps eliminate dandruff.

The other uncanny cosmetic effect of cider vinegar is that it relieves tiredness. Slowly massage it into the back neck, shoulders and arms, to cure body fatigue. Sometimes, after a tiring day hunched over the typewriter, I use this vinegar massage, then pop into a bath with vinegar and some anti-fatigue herbs (see Chapter III). If this doesn't do the trick (it usually does) I take a vitamin C tablet and a calcium tablet (dolomite plus magnesium), or a tablespoon of brewer's yeast, and in a short time I'm refreshed and full of energy.

You can use vinegar straight from the bottle on the face, but it is much wiser to *dilute* complexion vinegars about 8 to 1 with water or rose or orange water, especially if it is used often to reduce a tendency to skin oiliness. In an interesting 1890 manual, a doctor advises the use of such cosmetic vinegars but warns against using soap first, as the vinegar will decompose soap residues. I'm against using soap on the face anyway, as there are better, non-alkaline ways of cleansing the delicate skin on the face.

Aromatic Vinegars

Sweeter smelling, or cosmetic aromatic, vinegars can be created by adding to a bottle of cider or white vinegar, or for a tonic, wine vinegar, such dried or fresh herbs as lavender, violet, roses, rosemary; or oils of bergamot, lavender, rosemary, peppermint, verbena, carnation, rose geranium.

Lavender vinegar is my own favourite. It has been popular for thousands of years, and is described in one old manuscript thus: "It is cooling, and if the face is washed with it, it gives a firmness to and braces the fibres of the skin when too much relaxed."

Fresh Flower Vinegar

lavender flowers†	6 tablespoons
water	1 pint
cider or white vinegar	2 pints

Add lavender flowers to vinegar, steep for 2 weeks and add water.

† Or any aromatic flower.

Essence Vinegar

oil or essence of lavender‡	½ teaspoon
cider or white vinegar	1 pint
water	1 pint

Aromatic Tonic Vinegar

fresh rose petals*	1 ounce
white wine vinegar	¼ pint

Use a double boiler. Let rose petals and wine vinegar steep for 20 minutes in the upper half over the boiling water. Place in jar. Cover vinegar and roses with cloth or foil. Set in warm place. Steep 2 weeks. Strain petals from lotion. Place in tightly lidded jar.

15. NATURAL DEODORANTS

Children don't have a body odour—it is only with the onset of puberty and hormone production that our perspiration starts to have a strong smell. Chlorophyll, being bactericidal, has a marked effect on the bacteria which cause body odour, so if you eat foods rich in this substance, and use these chlorophyll herbs and foods on your body, you will be using helpful natural deodorants.

When the weather is hot, or when you are active, you will perspire more. This is the time to supplement our diet with food rich in nicotinic acid, one of the B vitamins, which you can find in peanuts, bran, mushrooms and brewer's yeast. Brewer's yeast is an excellent B supplement.

‡ Or any aromatic oil or essence.
* Or any aromatic flower petals.

Food Deodorants

All green leafy vegetables and some root tops are high in chlorophyll, and the ones that can be eaten, as well as rubbed under the armpits, to diminish perspiration odour, are parsley, watercress and the tops of beets, radish and turnip and the dark outside leaves of lettuce. Many people who try to eat less meat, or who eliminate meat entirely from their diet and eat a profusion of green vegetables, find that their perspiration doesn't have such a strong smell though they perspire just as much.

Herb, Oil, Flower Deodorants

There are several herbs, oils and flowers which can be helpful in controlling body odour. Those considered outstanding by the ancient herbalists are sage, lovage, cleavers, leaves of chrysanthemum, and oils of lavender, camphor and patchouli.

Sage is used by the Chinese in a strong infusion to control excessive perspiration odour, while lovage and cleavers are both drunk as a tea for this purpose, and used in strong infusion in the bath and under the armpits.

Lavender oil is an effective natural deodorant, but it is far too strong to use as an oil, except a drop at a time as a perfume. Make up a lavender water following the directions in Chapter X. It makes a delightful eau de cologne, and should be on everyone's shelf.

An anti-perspirant drink that has a valued reputation is one made of oil of camphor (BP), lemon and milk. Soak some lemon peel and fruit in warm milk and add 3 drops of camphor oil to the milk. Before retiring each night you can either drink the milk or chew the lemon rind.

Two young girls I know, who were allergic to every commercial deodorant they tried, used cider vinegar plus water and reported that it was very effective. The vinegar restores the skin to its normal pH value with its proper acid mantle, and although you still perspire there is far less odour. This treatment gets better as you use it. The smell of cider vinegar evaporates in about 10 minutes. See Section 14.

Patchouli oil and leaves and vetiver roots and oil are used by the Arabs in mattresses and pillows to suppress the smell of perspiration. The oil and essence as used in fragrances and soaps are said to have the same effect.

CHAPTER III

BATHING

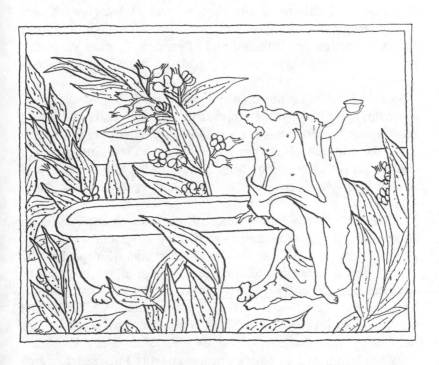

Many ancient cultures developed their social life and institutions around the idea of group bathing, and indeed the Japanese still have a form of family bathing. The ancient Assyrians restricted certain helpful herbs and oils to the royal family, and others to the nobles, while the less efficacious herbs were assigned to the common people. On the other hand, in Syria the King sometimes joined his subjects in the bathhouse. Antiochus was once accosted by one of his subjects while bathing with the words, "You must be a happy man, O King: you smell in a most *costly* manner!" Antiochus, far from being displeased, smilingly poured his expensive unguent over the man's head, while other poorer people crowded round to capture droplets of the precious oil. The Romans also went en masse to their elegant and beautiful marble bathhouses. In the famous Baths of Caracalla, considered the most beautiful of all the ancient bathhouses, up to 2,300 Roman citizens could choose from at least two dozen highly imaginative healthy and skin-restoring mineral, steam, massage, friction or oil baths, and often rich Romans vied with each other to see whose bath oil had the most interesting fragrance.

What has to be accepted in our own time is the versatility of the bath, for it is *not* just for cleansing. A bath can be extremely relaxing and soporific, or energizing and circulation-building. With the addition of certain herbs it can be soothing, healing, calming, reviving or stimulating. A bath can soften the skin and keep it from getting rough or brittle; it can replace lost moisture, oil and acidity.

Although we owe a deep debt of gratitude to the American Indian for his system of herbal medicine—a system we are just beginning to discover again—it is from the Europeans, the Asians and the peoples of the Near East that we inherit our bath cosmetic lore. There are dozens of stories about famous beauties and their favourite herbs: for instance, Catherine the Great was so involved with herbs, and what they could do for her beauty, that she created her own Russian "Pony Express," whose only job was to comb Europe and the Far East for aromatic and skin-nourishing plants. She took a long bath in these herbs every day, and once she tarried so long that she kept a great ambassador waiting for his audience. He was so outraged that it almost caused an international incident.

The French beauty Madame de Pompadour was the mistress of Louis XV of France and from the age of twenty-four until her death virtually ruled France. She was a friend of Voltaire and other authors of the *Encyclopédie,* and employed many artists to decorate her seven châteaux. However, La Pompadour was justifiably unpopular for her extravagance, which included a complete corps—almost an army—which did nothing but search for and collect herbs for her famous baths. Because bathing had fallen into disrepute during the Middle Ages and was not yet completely in favour, Louis XV asked his physicians to entreat his mistress not to take so many baths, fearing they would destroy her beauty, but La Pompadour ignored their advice and, it is said, used her herbs to great advantage.

Nowadays you don't need an army to gather and prepare herbs, for that has been done for you by the great botanical houses. In fact, you need only a postcard to ask for a catalogue and the world's exotic, natural substances become available to you immediately.

Basic Needs for Bathing

Although hot water is needed initially to release the essences and principles of the herbs, oils and foods suggested, you should never bathe in very hot water for a long time, as this de-energizes the body. Hot water is inadvisable for those with either sensitive, thin skins or thread veins on face or body.

For totally relaxing and soaking baths you should have a stretch-out tub; a non-slip mat or pasted non-slip strips, a large, comfortable rubber pillow to rest your head; and large, rough towels.

On the subject of towels, there is some interesting contradictory advice from an outstanding bath expert, the nineteenth-century herbalist, Father Kneipp. He suggested not using a towel but rather wrapping oneself into a rough cloth mantle or cotton robe, or immediately climbing into absorbent clothes and walking around or exercising until the body returned to its normal temperature.

To Read or Not to Read in the Bath

This must depend on your state of tiredness or your need to re-energize. If you want a truly relaxing bath, use the time to rest your eyes. An actress I know works very hard when she is in a film or on the stage and uses her bath-time to recharge. "I turn out all the lights except a small night light, allow some more warm water to flow into the bath, and in 15 minutes I feel revitalized," she says. "I find cucumber restful for my eyes, so while bathing, I often place a slice of cucumber on each eye, and gently palm each piece until the juice clears the eyes."

16. HERB BATHS

How to Use Herbs in the Bath

The only thing you must not do is just throw herbs *into* the bath. The smell is marvellous and they have a therapeutic effect of course; but if you try it, and I did, you will discover it takes about an hour to dislodge all the pieces of leaves, berries or bark from your body. So the thing to do is to use either a bath pochette or a strong herb infusion. Directions for infusion can be found in Chapter I.

You can make a bath pochette by enclosing your favourite herbs in a bag made of porous cloth, such as cheesecloth. For a more attractive effect, put the disposable cheesecloth bag in a patterned or colourful muslin or silk drawstring bag. These can be hung over the hot water tap and used for several consecutive baths, so it saves time and trouble to put together a pochette. A possible modern version which works well for me is one of those oval, stainless steel hinged tea containers for making individual cups of tea. Most of them have chains, and they can be tied to the hot water tap.

Two Versatile Herbs

Chamomile is a mild apple-smelling yellow and white flower. It is one of the most versatile of all herbs, and can be used in hair rinses, hair dyes, eye washes, facials. It contains azulene, a most soothing substance to the skin. Use the fresh leaves and flowers, or the dried flowers.

Since chamomile makes an excellent cleansing substance it is good for body care in the bath. For an extra fillip and a more stimulating action use ½ cup of chamomile with a dash of rosemary, horsetail and pine needles (or extract). During the summer when you are plagued by insect bites chamomile will protect you. Use in the bath; afterwards pat on a strong infusion of the flowers over all exposed parts of the body, and the insects will avoid you.

Elder leaves, berries, bark and flowers are considered healing for eyes; as an ointment, healing for sores of all kinds; and in infusion soothing for the nerves and helpful in falling asleep. In the bath elder can bleach, heal and stimulate the skin.

Aromatic Herbs

Every period of history has had its own attitude to bathing. In England in the seventeeth century perfumed baths came into favour, and roses, lemon flowers, jasmine, bay, lavender, mint, pennyroyal and citron peel were used alone or together with a few drops of oil of spike and some fixative such as musk or ambergris. It is quite simple to obtain these oils and essences today, and you can certainly combine them for your aromatic baths.

Lovage is not a highly aromatic herb, but it has the virtue of being both cleansing and deodorant. It is a member of the parsley family; and parsley, as you may recall, can even erase the smell of onions and garlic on the breath. Gently boil the lovage root for 20 minutes. Strain and use. For more on natural deodorants, see Section 15.

Healing Herbs

There are many healing herbs, but not all lend themselves to infusion and use in the bath. Of the several that I would recommend, *comfrey* is perhaps the most helpful and important, as it is an all-round healing herb. Because of its power to help mend fractured bones, country folk call it "knit-bone." The leaves can make a valuable poultice for all kinds of sores, burns, swellings, and can be used in strong infusion in the bath water. The roots, too, release a large amount of mucilage which is easily extracted by hot water.

Lady's mantle, a delightful pleated herb (hence the name), is valued by the Arabs for all kinds of women's troubles. It can help heal inflammations and even acne.

Marigold leaves also have a reputation for healing, and under its other name, calendula, it can be found in many ointments. The leaves can be used in tepid baths since they have a reputation for helping those with body scars and thread veins, and of soothing those with varicose veins.

The Latin name for yarrow is *Achillea millefolium.* The herb is a useful and powerful astringent, and therefore is of special interest to those with excess oil on their face and body since it can be used in the bath, in an infusion as a facial ingredient, and internally as a tea. When used as a tea it can bring on perspiration and thus cleanse the system. If you feel an illness coming on drink a strong infusion with equal parts of yarrow, peppermint and elder flower. Hop into bed and go to sleep. You will feel much better when you awaken. A yarrow compress can also alleviate soreness of the nipples.

Linden (*lime*) and *nettle* leaves contain a compound physiologically related to natural hormones, and are helpful for body skin. In addition, nettles contain the vitamins A and C. *Dandelions* also have many plant hormones and can be combined with nettles for a most cleansing and helpful bath.

Mint has healing properties and can be used in the bath to heal minor skin eruptions.

Houseleek has always been considered a valuable skin herb, and can be used for healing and nourishing baths.

The famous French beauty Ninon de Lenclos, who remained unwrinkled and youthful-looking to a great old age, was exceptionally fond of houseleek in her creams and facials. It is said that her secret bath herbs were a combination of houseleek, mint, lavender, thyme and rosemary.

Nourishing Baths

Have you ever noticed that many people pay attention to their face—in the sense that they cream it and use many nourishing products—but never think of using restoring products on their body through massage creams and bath oils? The body skin can dry out too and lose its resilience and disease-resistant acid mantle; so it is very important to know the ingredients which can soothe, replenish and nourish.

Many beauty experts advise using both almond oil and avocado oil in nourishing home baths since these oils also have vitamins that are useful to the body. Lisa Kosman, who manages the "Good Earth," New York's largest health food supermarket, told me that she often uses a dollop of sunflower or sesame seed oil in her bath to replace outer body oils.

Herbal Bath Oils

Dispersing oil is one that completely dissolves in water. There are very few of these, but the oil of the castor plant can, when treated, be an ideal bath oil, as it dissolves completely and does not leave a ring. Treated castor oil is known as Turkey-red oil.

Turkey-red oil	¾ cup
aromatic oil	¼ cup

Mix together. Bottle. Label. Use 1 teaspoon per bath.

Floating oil is one that is lighter than water and floats on top. It will cling to your skin as you emerge from the bath. Almond oil and avocado oil are such oils.

almond oil	¾ cup
aromatic oil	¼ cup
or, an alternative recipe	
almond oil	½ cup
avocado oil	¼ cup
aromatic oil	¼ cup

Mix together. Bottle. Label. Use 1 teaspoon per bath.

Any of these oils will cost far less and be far purer than most commercially available bath capsules. With a little experimentation, particularly with different scents, you should be able to make up bath oils for yourself and your family, and as gifts for friends.

Herbal Oil Soap

chamomile	2 tablespoons
(or nettle, lime flower, elder flower, fennel)	
milk	12 tablespoons
egg	1
almond oil	8 tablespoons
herbal shampoo	2 tablespoons
honey	1 teaspoon
(or coconut oil shampoo or castile shampoo)	
isopropyl alcohol	2 tablespoons
(or perfume)	

Drench chamomile (or other suggested herb) in the cold milk and let it stand with a porous cover for 3 hours. Strain. Discard chamomile flowers. Put herb-milk aside. Mix the egg with the almond oil and beat until entirely smooth. Add and keep mixing the shampoo, and as you keep beating also add the honey and isopropyl rubbing alcohol. Blend in the herb-milk. Pour into a labelled jar. This needs frequent shaking, but is a useful and effective bath oil soap. Should you decide to make it up in larger quantities, keep it in the refrigerator.

For a more aromatic effect, cut oil to 6 tablespoons and add combination of 1 tablespoon oil of lavender, ½ tablespoon of oil of lemon, ¼ tablespoon of oil of cloves.

For increased stimulation from this bath oil soap, particularly in the case of body aches, add ¼ teaspoon of either oil of pine or oil of eucalyptus to the original recipe.

17. SOOTHING AND TONING BATHS

Oatmeal, Almond Meal, Cornmeal, Bran Baths

When I was a child we always used leftover oatmeal for night-time baths since oatmeal is exceptionally cleansing and soothing to the body, can heal inflamed skin and keep it milky white.

A modern oatmeal bath can be made with colloidal oatmeal, which can be kept in its own container in the bathroom. Plaster a dampened handful all over your body, and throw another handful into the bath under the running water—it will disperse. Remove the body "mask" with a friction glove or a loofah.

Do the same with paste made of almond meal, or cornmeal, or bran and water.

Milk Baths

Many beauties of the past, including Cleopatra, were known for their extravagant milk baths. Milk is an extremely nourishing, soothing substance and will help smooth the skin and give it a lustrous finish. It is healing for roughened skin. Tepid milk baths (or facials) are helpful both for acne and for black-heads (see Section 5).

For additional softening power in a milk bath, add a strong infusion of elder flower or chamomile, or nettle, or lime flower (linden).

George Sand's Replenishing Milk Bath

When the Baroness Aurore Dudevant left her husband and went to live and work with the writer Jules Sandeau, she changed her name to George Sand. She earned her living, and supported her children, by writing; some of her eighty novels are certainly autobiographical, and describe her liaisons with, among others, the poet Alfred de Musset and the composer Chopin. Apparently George Sand wasn't beautiful, but she had lovely, alive-looking skin which she took care to preserve. She used milk, honey, salt and bicarbonate of soda in her bath.

The salt can remove toxins and dead skin cells, and the honey and milk are softeners. If you like you can leave out the bicarbonate of soda, and you will need to scale the quantities down, but here I give the original recipe.

Dissolve 3½ ounces of bicarbonate of soda and 8 ounces of kitchen salt in a quart of water. Dissolve 3 pounds of honey in 3 quarts of milk. Pour the soda and salt solution into the bath, mix and stir in the milk and honey.

Expensive Baths

There were several famous beauties who had nightly baths in berries—some used strawberries, other raspberries. Isabelle of Bavaria took spring and summer baths in strawberry juice. Strawberries, of course, are delightfully cooling and cleansing to the skin, and they have internal cleansing power too. Another famous beauty, Madam Tallien, favoured a bath of crushed strawberries and raspberries, after which she was gently rubbed with sponges soaked in perfumed milk. Mary Queen of Scots preserved her beauty by bathing in wine, a habit which the Earl of Shewsbury, in whose charge she was, found so costly that he had to ask the government to increase his allowance for taking care of the Queen.

Tonic Spring Baths

Everyone who lives in a cold winter climate longs for a tonic spring bath to brighten dingy winter skin. If you are lucky enough to know where there are unsprayed blackberry leaves, collect and crush them and add boiling water to make an especially strong infusion. These blackberry leaves are particularly effective if used several nights in a row in your bath water. Your skin will have a new look and glow.

Friction Baths

The body is constantly renewing its cells and actually replaces all of them in a seven-year period. Wherever you increase your circulation with exercise, towelling, salt, oil or loofah or brush rubs, you are aiding the process of replacement, and you will look and feel far better.

Circulation Baths

The famous mineral and ocean spas provide excellent circulation baths. It is hard to obtain the special mineral mud from mineral spas, but you will find it quite simple to make your own circulation bath. Combine ½ pound of magnesium sulphate (epsom salts) and 1 pound of magnesium chloride in your warm bath. If you want to have a health-giving touch and an invigorative smell add eucalyptus, pine or mint extract or oil. If you want to use your own pine needles, either boil them for 20 minutes or place them in a large thermos flask, pour boiling water over them, let them steep for 12 to 24 hours, and strain and use a cupful at a time.

Salt Toner Rub

If you are feeling particularly sluggish and want to tone up your body, you can also take a sea salt, or coarse salt, or epsom salt rub *before* this spa bath. A doctor once explained to me that epsom salts removes toxicity from the body. None of these salts should be used too often, however.

The salt should be slightly moistened and rubbed, half a handful at a time, over the shoulders and arms, and then over the rest of the body, omitting the genital area and the face. Stand in the bath. Take a "circulation" or ordinary warm bath. Add a restoring oil to the water or rub it on your body. Incidentally, don't forget to rinse the salt carefully out of the bath, as it can corrode metal and porcelain.

Cider Vinegar Bath or Rub

One of the simplest and most effective baths is one to which you add one cup of cider vinegar, which restores the acid mantle to the skin. If you are feeling very tired, you can also dilute the vinegar with 8 parts of water and rub it on your body before stepping into the bath. It takes away any itchiness, flakiness and dryness of the skin.

Toning Baths

For an immediate refreshing pick up, try the *cold* friction bath. Dip your body into cold water and rub yourself all over with a loofah or a rough flannel. Do this for only a few minutes and get out, and either towel yourself dry or get into absorbent clothes and exercise until your temperature returns to normal.

Alternating hot and cold foot baths or general body baths are very stimulating to the body and should be taken whenever you feel fatigued and want an immediate lift. This effect can be increased by standing under a warm shower and using a cold shower spray from another tap on your body—feeling the two temperatures at the same time.

Cold knee baths, either sitz baths in cold water or kneeling baths in cold water, are very stimulating to the system and may be used just before going to sleep to aid sleep, or first thing in the morning to revive the body. This might sound contradictory but it really works very well.

Cold foot baths: stand in cold water up to your calves for one to three minutes—very stimulating and reviving for the body. This, like the knee baths, can help you sleep, or revive you in the morning.

CHAPTER IV

HAIR

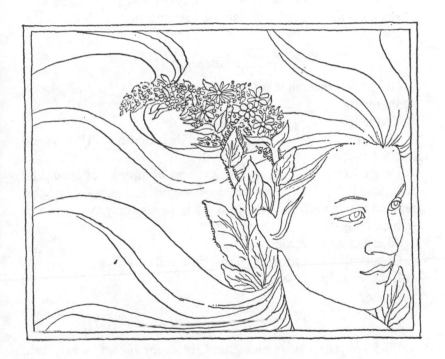

Hair is a fairly good indicator of general health, as are the complexion, clearness of the eyes and colour and quality of the fingernails. It is one of the doctor's instant indicators of negative or positive health.

Like the outer covering on our body and fingernails, hair is a form of skin—a protein actually—called keratin. It gets its nourishment from the food we eat, and therefore fairly quickly indicates either the lack of nutrients, or often, the lack of absorption of specific foods. Most adults have about 100,000 hairs growing on their heads, and these can survive for between two years and ten, depending on age, race and sex.

It is generally agreed that heredity, food, moisture, protein and oils are the biggest factors in hair health. Undoubtedly, if you have parents or grandparents who have strong or healthy hair, you should too. That is, barring accidents, serious infections and a period of unusual strain or tension, since these and lack of sleep greatly affect the growth of hair and the way it looks.

Hair Enemies

Overindulgence in carbohydrates, empty dry cereals, cake, soda, sugar.

Too much sun.

Nylon brushes (they split ends and damage hair). Use natural bristle brush.

Drugs. Prescription drugs in the form of antibiotics should be accompanied by a cup or more of yogurt a day, as this helps replace the "good" bacteria your body needs for proper absorption and digestion.

Allergies and infection.

Chemicals in the form of rinses, tints and bleaches.

Lack of scalp massage.

Food for the Hair

Whether your hair is blond, red, black or brown, shiny, dull, dry or oily, it will respond to intelligent and thoughtful food nurturing. Some nutritionists consider brewer's yeast and liver the hair-restoring foods, and suggest careful examination of one's daily diet to check that enough B complex, A and C and calcium foods are taken, as well as the "hair" minerals, iron, iodine and copper.

Of the minerals, lack of iodine is the most damaging, as it normally supplies the thyroid gland and helps with scalp circulation. If the circulation in the scalp is too slow it soon shows in extremely dull hair which falls out. If you are combing out huge clumps of hair you probably need professional help with this problem. As I have mentioned, if you are ill or not eating correctly your system removes the necessary nutrients from your nails, skin, teeth and hair to feed the more important functioning organs. Since brewer's yeast is an excellent B complex supplement, take up to 3 to 5 tablespoons a day for real hair troubles.

Other important foods for hair restoring are green salads and fresh raw vegetables, particularly watercress, white part of leeks, carrots and potatoes, fruits, particularly apples and oranges. Fresh fish and some sea vegetation, liver twice a week, raisins and polyunsaturated oils like safflower (or sunflower, soy, wheat germ, corn or olive in that order) are also a necessary part of the diet.

18. SCALP EXERCISES

The best way to increase the circulation of your scalp is to learn the yoga headstand and do it every day. If this is too difficult, the next best thing is the preparatory posture—the shoulder stand which is much easier. Lie on your back, then raise your body and rest it on your shoulders and elbows. Keep your feet high and legs straight. You will feel the chest pressing on the neck and the thyroid gland, and this helps to activate it.

The following is a head massage which you can practise any time of the day.

Curl up each hand as though you were grasping a rather slippery orange, so that your fingers are tensed and strong. With the cushion of each of your ten tensed fingers, press down in a circular motion until you feel the warmth of the blood rushing to the area. Then move on to another spot on the scalp until your whole head is tingling and alive. Alternatively, you can use a small hand vibrator.

19. SHAMPOOING

You can make a herbal shampoo by adding a strong infusion of herbs to your favourite coconut, castile or avocado shampoo. Also, you can add these herbs to a plant substance containing nature's soaping ingredient—saponin.

For a *light hair* shampoo, make a strong chamomile infusion and add to shampoo. Besides being a hair lightener, chamomile is a softening agent.

Add an infusion of mullein flowers or nettle, or a decoction of rhubarb root.

Those with normal or oily light hair can add a beaten egg white; those with dry light hair a beaten egg yolk.

For a *dark hair* shampoo, add either rosemary or sage infusion, or rosemary oil. These herbs revitalize hair.

Dry Shampooing

In many parts of the world, particularly the Far East where the women and men pride themselves on their long, lustrous and healthy hair, few people ever *wash* the hair. Instead they brush through it some form of absorbent meal or powder, depending on available resources. In India, for instance, those who follow the old ways use a form of cornmeal and brush it through the hair until it is clean. The advantage of these dry shampoos is the sparkling look they give to the hair once they are properly brushed out, and the boost the hair gets when its necessary 2 per cent acid mantle is not constantly washed out.

Orrisroot from pulverized Florentine iris root has been used for dry shampoos for many centuries. Fuller's earth can also be used.

Part the hair in sections and sprinkle in the absorbent substance until the whole head has been covered at the scalp. Brush vigorously 5 minutes later.

Another dry shampoo is the following which I picked up from my husband, who in his work as a stage and film make-up man is often forced to work under rigorous location difficulties. "When there is absolutely no time or place to wash a head of hair," he says, "I suggest that the actor or actress cover a brush and force the bristles through a piece of cheesecloth or nylon. Sprinkle the cloth with eau de cologne, and brush through the hair. A surprising amount of dust and grey dirt will adhere to the cloth. This can be thrown away and the same process repeated if there is more dirt in the hair."

20. CONDITIONERS

If you don't have lustrous hair, you need a conditioner. To condition hair properly, wash it first with a herbal shampoo. Add conditioner-treatment anything from 15 minutes to several hours later. Rinse out the conditioner. Set or dry the hair.

Hot Oil

You can use very warm olive oil as a weekly conditioner. Other possible oils are castor oil, which is very strengthening, and such penetrating oils as almond and avocado. Safflower and corn oil will also do.

Heat the oil and saturate the hair. Cover the hair with a layer of wax paper. Cover it again with a heavy-duty plastic cap. Add heat with an electric heat cap or heavy towel. These oils can also be left on overnight with good results.

Protein Treatments

Eggs contain one of the best proteins for the hair. They are full of lecithin, which is very helpful in restoring hair texture and tone.

Protein Cure

The following treatment combines protein, emollients and lecithin, all of which are helpful to brittle hair:

lanolin	3 tablespoons
castor oil	3 tablespoons
olive oil	¼ cup
liquid castile soap	1 tablespoon
glycerine	4 tablespoons
water	1¼ cups
egg yolk	2 tablespoons
cider vinegar	1 teaspoon
eggs	2

optional

perfume essence	10 drops

In the top of a double boiler blend together lanolin, castor oil and olive oil. Turn off the heat for at least 5 minutes and let the blended oils sit. Slowly, with an electric mixer, stir in liquid castile soap, glycerine and water. Use a low speed until the mixture thickens. With the beater on high add 2 tablespoons of beaten egg yolk, cider vinegar, and 10 drops of your favourite pure perfume essence. Pour into a jar and label, and refrigerate for several hours or overnight. The next day add 2 eggs on high speed. Refrigerate leftovers.

Quick Protein Cure

eggs	1 or 2 (depending on hair brittleness)
castor oil (or wheat germ, olive, corn, safflower oil)	1 tablespoon 1 tablespoon
glycerine	1 teaspoon
cider vinegar	

Beat together all ingredients. Apply after initial shampoo. Leave on for at least 15 minutes to ½ hour. Rinse.

Cocoa Butter Conditioner

This is almost the same cocoa butter recipe as you use for dry skin cleansing and care, but here safflower oil is preferred.

safflower oil	½ cup
cocoa butter	1 tablespoon
anhydrous lanolin	1 tablespoon

In the top of a double boiler melt together the oil, the cocoa butter and the lanolin until they are *completely* dissolved and blended together. Beat with an electric mixer. Take about 3 tablespoons of above mixture and add 1 tablespoon of water. Mix again. Label the jar as cocoa butter conditioner. Use on hair if it is very dry.

Parsnip Conditioner

This is vouched for by a lady whose great-great-grandmother passed it on to her:

Simmer together 1 chopped parsnip root, ½ teaspoon of parsnip seeds and ¼ cup of olive oil (or *any* of the previously mentioned oils). Steep for ½ hour. Strain and use on hair.

21. DRY HAIR

Occasionally people ask me to tell them whether they have dry hair, as they aren't sure. Well, if it looks dry to you, feels less than soft and lacks *lustre,* it is dry. The first positive step you can take in restoring your hair and making it more beautiful, and rescuing it from dryness, is elimination of most sugar products, since they destroy B vitamins, and you need Bs for lustrous hair.

Shampooing Dry Hair

Shampoo no more than once a week. First wash your hair with a restorative herbal shampoo. (If it is especially limp add a whole beaten egg, or preferably 2 egg yolks and ½ packet of unflavoured gelatine dissolved in ¼ cup of boiling water.) Condition your hair—see Section 20. Rinse out the conditioner.

People with dry hair must follow this sequence exactly. Always condition the hair *after* you wash it, and just rinse out the conditioner. In this way you do not neutralize or cancel out the effects of the conditioner.

Restoring Lustre

Rosemary is particularly good for people with dark hair. Oil of rosemary untangles hard-to-manage hair and adds sheen.

rosemary	2 tablespoons
boiling water	1 pint
oil of sweet almonds	3 ounces
lavender essence	30 drops

Mix together 1 ounce of an infusion of rosemary and almond oil and lavender to create a scented lustre-restorer for dark hair.

Parsley can also be used. Boil it in water for 20 minutes. Use water as a final rinse to add sheen to hair.

22. OILY HAIR

Although oily hair seems harder to manage than dry hair, it can be brought back to normal with proper diet, consistent and careful brushing, scalp massage and exercise. Excess oil in the hair means that the sebaceous glands of your scalp are far too active, and you should immediately cut down on animal fats and fried foods in your diet. Occasionally, too, oily hair is a result of poor thyroid function and stress. If you suspect either, you should see your doctor.

Anti-strain Relaxer

One exercise which stimulates the thyroid is the following anti-strain relaxer, which increases the circulation to your shoulders and neck:

Lie on your back with your palms up and rest for a few minutes. Close your eyes. Your body should feel heavy. Clench your left hand. Lift it, tense it hard. Let it fall limply so that all tension disappears. Do this for your right hand. Lift and tense your left leg, then let it fall limply. Same for the other leg. Then grimace. Make a tense, sour face. Stick out your tongue, push out your eyes. Let your face relax. Starting with your toes and concentrating on each part of your body, force yourself to relax until you are completely limp and relaxed. Lie like this for as long as you wish.

Then *lift your head* up until your chin is resting on your neck. Do this several times. This encourages thyroid activity. So does the *shoulder stand*. Lift your entire body up until it rests on your elbows and feel the pressure of the thyroid on the chest. This exercise is excellent for everybody and will help revitalize hair and skin.

Food for Oily Hair

Foods rich in iodine and food with high B complex factors are helpful in eliminating oily hair. Soybeans, soy sauce, seaweed and kelp are also helpful. Drink yarrow or lady's mantle tea several times a day. Add yarrow infusion to your shampoo. Use frequent cider vinegar rinses after shampoo—½ cup to a quart of water.

Oily Hair Shampoos

Shampoo often, even once a day.

Dark-haired people with oily hair should use the following herbs added to castile or other herbal shampoos.

Make a decoction of 1 tablespoon of southernwood, 1 tablespoon of quassia chips. Simmer together in 1 pint of water for 20 minutes. Add a teaspoon of rosemary. Steep for another 3 minutes. Cool. Strain and add to shampoo.

Another drying shampoo which also restores lustre and body to the hair is the following:

whole eggs	4
rum	1 cup
rose water	1 cup

Beat eggs and massage through hair. Wash off 15 minutes later. Rinse with equal parts of rum and rose water.

If you can't wash your hair every day, an orrisroot, or fuller's earth *dry* shampoo is very effective, as is the nylon- or cheesecloth-covered hair brush to remove dirt and grime. Oily hair responds to vigorous and constant brushing.

23. FINAL RINSES

Vinegar

Cider vinegar is a very old rinse and would benefit most people since it helps restore the acid covering that has just been washed away with the shampoo. It also removes the last vestiges of soap in the hair. It must be diluted in rinse water (see Section 14).

Dark Hair Rinses

A rinse to add lustre to dark hair could include southernwood and quassia chips boiled gently for 15 minutes. Use 1 teaspoon of southernwood to 2 tablespoons of quassia chips to a pint of water. Steep for ½ hour, strain and use to bring out the natural highlights of dark hair.

Rosemary is another excellent rinse ingredient for dark-haired people. Use 2 tablespoons to a pint of boiling water. Steep and strain. Add to final rinse water.

Light Hair Rinses

Light brown and blond hair will respond to chamomile or mullein flowers or rhubarb root infusions added to final rinse water. Lemon or cider vinegar can also be added to the final rinse. For a thorough discussion of these see Section 28.

24. NATURAL SETTING LOTIONS

There are a great many natural substances which can easily be added to shampoos and rinses, or which can be used as a *setting lotion* for hair which hangs too limp and straight. While it is true these home products take a bit more time to make than shop items, they give a boost to the hair and do not leave any dry, flaky residue.

Rosemary

Rosemary is one of the best herbs for the hair and can be used in massages, rinses and shampoos as well as setting lotions. According to Dr. Fernie, the author of *Herbal Simples,* written several hundred years ago, you could do no better than wash or rinse your hair in rosemary. He recommends it particularly for rainy days. "It has the singular power," he writes, "of preventing the hair from *uncurling* when exposed to a damp atmosphere." Fernie's recipe consists of an infusion of rosemary—2 tablespoons or 1 ounce to a pint of boiling water. Steep for a few hours, strain and use either in shampoo or final rinse water.

Another version of this tonic is rosemary and equal parts of sage combined. Prepare the same way as above. Both these herbs are best for people with dark brown or black hair.

Quince, Flaxseed, Irish Moss and Gums

Nature has provided us with many natural setting lotions. Quince seed is one of the very best. Simmer a teaspoon in boiling water until the mixture thickens. For a longer lasting quince seed setting lotion add a tablespoon of eau de cologne to each tablespoon of dissolved seed. Quince is also a known hair reviver.

Flaxseed (linseed) and Irish moss (carragheen) also add body to the hair. To use them dissolve a tablespoon at a time in a tablespoon of boiling water until the mixture thickens.

Dissolve any of the gums in the same way. Use either gum tragacanth, gum arabic or gum acacia.

The following recipe can be used with any of the above herbs, although gum tragacanth is listed:

water	¾ cup
gum tragacanth	1 teaspoon
ethyl rubbing alcohol (buy best brand)	¼ cup
glycerine	3 drops
perfume (optional)	3 drops

Boil water in double boiler and stir gum tragacanth on the surface of the water. Do not let powder (or herbs) go lumpy. Add the alcohol, glycerine, perfume. Stir again. Stand overnight to thicken.

For a thicker lotion lessen the water and alcohol. For a thinner lotion increase alcohol. The thinned version can be used in an atomizer.

Gelatine

Natural gelatine can also be used as a gelling agent for setting hair, or as a hair body builder for limp or thin hair. For a hair thickening effect, use a packet of the dissolved gelatine plus a whole egg and herbal shampoo. Wash hair with mixture.

Gelatine can also be added to rinse water to increase the heaviness of the hair. Coloured gelatines can be used in the following way: lemon for light hair; raspberry, strawberry or cherry for redheads and brunettes. The sugar in the coloured gelatines seems to add additional body, in the same way that sugar in the final rinse water adds body (almost like a starch) to fabrics.

Lemon Hair-setting Lotion

Another excellent hair-setting lotion was discovered by my husband while he was working on make-up with some film stars. Many actresses use lemon juice to set their hair. This takes a long time to dry, but it has the advantage of holding the set for a long time. You can use bottled lemon juice or make a better, thicker, faster drying, whole-lemon version. Either squeeze the juice of several lemons in a juice extractor and strain and use, or chop up some lemons, boil them in water and strain when the juice seems reduced. For the fresh lemon version, add a teaspoon of eau de cologne as lemon attracts mould. Otherwise keep in the refrigerator.

25. TONICS

Hair is a reflection of the whole person, and if your spirits are low or you have been deprived of adequate food or sleep this will show up in the form of dull, listless and sometimes falling hair. Brushing should be the first order of attack. Make sure you have a natural-bristle brush and spend that old-fashioned 100 strokes a night on *each section* of your hair. You will see results in a short time.

Under various other headings I have discussed the herbs and combinations which will help revitalize the hair. They are rosemary, sage, nettle, chamomile, castor oil and forms of gum camphor, as well as other stimulating herbs which are listed in various other recipes. For dark hair rosemary and sage are good tonic herbs; chamomile is best for light hair.

To make a hair tonic with herbs pour a pint of boiling water over 4 tablespoons of your chosen herb. Steep for several hours. Strain. To preserve this lotion add a few drops of eau de cologne or a dozen drops of gin. Either massage through hair, or use in shampoo or rinse water.

We discovered one of my grandmother's hair-reviving tonics in a book of her poems. It was the kind of recipe family friends frequently requested. Jaborandi is a stimulating herb. Use only *ethyl* rubbing alcohol, or a strong-proof vodka.

jaborandi	1 ounce
nettle	1 ounce
rosemary	1 ounce
ethyl alcohol (or vodka)	6 ounces
castor oil	12 drops
perfume	5 drops
salicylic acid	¼ ounce
distilled water	4 ounces

Soak jaborandi, nettle, rosemary in the alcohol for 3 weeks. Strain into another container. Add castor oil and perfume. Dissolve salicylic acid in distilled water. Add to herbal and oil solution. Use as a nightly massage.

Another hair-reviving herb is gum camphor. Steep 1 ounce of crushed gum camphor and 2 ounces of powdered borax in 2 quarts of boiling water for several hours. Massage nightly into hair and scalp.

26. DANDRUFF

To have a few of the white-flaked cells we call dandruff is normal, for it is simply the sloughing off of matured skin cells and food waste through the pores of the scalp. It is only when this becomes excessive that it has to be considered a problem. Well-brushed, clean, *healthy* hair with the proper balance of acid doesn't have problem dandruff.

There are two forms of dandruff, one oily and one dry, and the oily form is found most often among adolescents and adults with an excessively oily skin and scalp. According to the New York dermatologist Dr. Irwin Lubowe, the "basic causes of dandruff are faulty diet, emotional tension, hormonal disturbances, infection due to disease, injury to the scalp and unwise or excessive use of hair cosmetics." According to Dr. Lubowe, the reason why so many adolescents have dandruff is that this is the time when they secrete an excess of androgen hormones which cause sebum, the skin oil. To control dandruff many dermatologists and nutritionists therefore recommend the same restrictions on food that are listed for acne. Eat less animal fat, and more polyunsaturated vegetable oils and no nuts, chocolate, butter or fried foods, shellfish, iodized salt. A diet high in greens and first-class proteins and foods high in vitamins A, E and B complex are necessary.

Brushing

Vigorous, daily brushing is important in ridding the hair of dandruff and increasing circulation of the scalp.

Shampoos

Use herbal or castile shampoos and avoid all synthetic preparations for dandruff, some of which use too powerful drugs. Many are simply irritants which temporarily remove the dandruff, but most cause the scalp to produce more oil to protect itself. Some hairdressers tell me that the side effects of some of the dandruff remedies on the market are falling hair, excessive oiliness and allergic reaction. Some chemical hair sprays also *cause* flakiness and dandruff.

Vinegar

One of the quickest dandruff removers (and all who used it said itching of the scalp disappeared at the same time, too) is cider vinegar. It can be used diluted in water, and most particularly in lavender water, or other aromatic dilutions as a nightly massage. There is a description of vinegars in Section

14. Incidentally, if you should decide to use plain cider vinegar and water, be assured that the smell soon disappears.

Oil

Another easy home remedy is a treatment with hot castor oil (which strengthens the hair) or hot olive oil, or hot linseed oil (the kind you get from a health food store). Massage the hot oil into your hair for a twice-a-week treatment until you are rid of the dandruff. This is an excellent treatment for dry hair too.

After massaging your hair with the oil, put on a plastic heat cap, or shower cap plus towel, over the hair for about ½ hour. I prefer the electric heat cap as it shows immediate results. Since such a treatment is expensive in a beauty parlour, you can make up for your investment in this electric cap within 2 or 3 sessions.

Shampoo with non-detergent shampoo having either an olive oil, coconut, castile or avocado base.

Nettle

Of all the traditional herbal remedies nettle juice was the most acclaimed for hair treatment and is considered particularly effective for dandruff. Make your own strong infusion by adding a pint of boiling water to 4 tablespoons of nettle leaves and allowing to steep several hours. Add ¼ cup of cider vinegar and ¼ cup of eau de cologne to the strained nettle juice to make it last longer. Massage into scalp nightly. If your hair is very oily you can increase the amount of eau de cologne to ½ cup.

Rosemary

Rosemary tonic, as we have mentioned before, revives hair, gives it body and helps prevent it from uncurling. It also gives lustre to the hair and rids it of dandruff. No wonder most of the ancient herbal books rave about rosemary.

Combined with a pinch of borax, rosemary is considered by some herbalists to be one of the finest hair washes known. Rosemary and sage infusion can be used together, as they both have a stimulating effect on the hair. Massage through hair or use in shampoo or final rinse water.

Other Dandruff Chasers

There are many other dandruff chasers. For new cases, massage each night with witch hazel or lemon juice or rose water or willow-bark tea.

A combination of a tablespoon of eau de cologne and a pinch of borax is also useful.

27. HAIR GROWTH

The herbals are full of suggestions for increasing hair growth, but remember that only some forms of baldness are reversible. I met a young man recently who *had* reversed the process with scalp exercises, daily rests with his feet higher than his head, change of food habits to include huge amounts of vitamins (more on that later) and a shift from ordinary food to insecticide-free food. After being totally bald, in 3 months there was fuzz on his head and at the end of 8 months he had long hair in many areas of the head, and was still growing new baby soft hair in others.

Peter Flesch (in *Physiology and Biochemistry of the Skin*) mentions that many doctors have recorded good results from the use of pantothenic acid, and describes a German experiment on a hypothyroid child whose "scant hair could not be restored by thyroid medication, even though other symptoms of hypothyroidism were alleviated. Administration of pantothenic acid brought about a dense growth of scalp hair."

Quince is used by the Arabs to increase the growth of the manes and tails of their beautiful horses.

Other useful herbs mentioned in old herbals and family recipe books are mallow roots, maidenhair fern spores, nettles, parsley seed, jaborandi, rosemary, boxwood shavings, nutmeg, willow leaves, cloves, artichokes.

The mallows may be boiled in wine and used as a massage. Maidenhair spores are boiled in wine in strong decoction; add white wine and massage through the hair. The parsley seeds are crushed and applied in powder form to the scalp once a month. Allow to remain overnight and brush out thoroughly.

The nettle infusion, or pure plant juice, can be combed through the hair, using an opposite stroke to natural direction of hair growth. Use daily if you can.

Jaborandi is used after infusion for 24 hours and combed through the hair.

In *The Art of Cookery Made Plain & Easy,* by a Lady, 1760, occurs the following note:

An Approved Method Practiced by Mrs Dukeley,
The Queen's Tyre Woman,
to Preserve Hair and Make it Grow Thick.

Take one quart of white wine, put in one handful of rosemary flowers, half a pound of honey, distill together; then add a quarter of a pint of oil of sweet almonds, shake it very well together, put a little of it into a cup, warm it blood warm, rub it well in your head and comb it dry.

Baron Dupuytren's Hair Growth Pomade

The baron gained world-wide fame for this pomade, which he claimed overcame baldness:

rosemary spirits	2 ounces
nutmeg spirits	½ ounce
ethyl alcohol	12 ounces
(or vodka)	
boxwood shavings	6 ounces

You can obtain spirits at the chemists, or you can make your own by submerging each of the herbs separately in some ethyl alcohol for about 10 days and straining off and using the alcohol. Steep boxwood shavings in alcohol or vodka for 2 weeks. Strain. Add rosemary spirits and nutmeg spirits. Massage into scalp every morning and evening.

Willow Fern Tonic

willow leaves	4 tablespoons
maidenhair fern	4 tablespoons
cloves	3
salad oil	2 cups
(or castor oil)	

Simmer together in the top of a double boiler for 1 hour. Turn off flame. Stand for another hour. Strain and pour into labelled bottle. This can be used nightly.

Artichoke Lotion

This was passed on to me by Monsieur Antoine Millet of Paris who told me the country people used this easy formula against baldness.

Simmer a dozen artichoke leaves in a cup of water for several hours. Use unstrained liquid as nightly massage.

Catnip

Catnip was used by many European gypsies in their rinse water to increase hair growth and eliminate scalp irritation leading to baldness.

28. HAIR COLOURING

There are many proven natural methods of changing hair colour or eliminating grey. Some have been passed down through the centuries. But before we consider these age-old, non-synthetic methods, let us look into modern scientific literature on colouring grey hair through vitamin supplements.

There have been many experiments, particularly with the so-called anti-grey vitamins, PABA (para-aminobenzoic acid), calcium pantothenate, choline and inositol, and although thousands of people now use these products and claim they help, legal restrictions on vouching for such vitamin therapy are so stringent that no reliable vitamin producer will allow himself to be quoted on this subject at this time, although privately they admit they have seen results.

Dr. Carlton Fredricks advises using these vitamins in a strong B complex base and also eating milk, brewer's yeast, whole wheat, whole rye, shellfish such as oysters, clams, shrimps and meats such as liver, sweetbreads, pork and ham. He warns that it will take a while to achieve results. PABA had been used in two experiments by Dr. Benjamin Sieve of Boston on patients who had had *grey* hair from 2 to 24 years. In 3 to 8 weeks the 800 grey-haired patients who were given this vitamin showed hair changes. Those who had had light hair before they were grey now had dirty-yellowish hair, and those who had dark hair before they were grey found that their hair changed to a darker, dusty greyish colour. While these particular experiments are not conclusive, they indicate that PABA may have an effect on grey hair.

Other suggestions from nutritionists include drinking a mixture of 2 tablespoons each of cider vinegar, uncooked honey and blackstrap molasses in a glass of water. This can be taken every morning on getting up. It is also re-energizing to the system.

Plant and Vegetable Hair Colouring

Most of the dyes on the markets today are aniline, which is a coal-tar product. Peter Morell, in *Poisons, Potions and Profits,* says, "Hair dyes probably lead the list as the most dangerous of all widely used cosmetics. Aniline dyes can be very injurious to those who are sensitive to such chemicals, and the damage may be of such varied nature that it would be difficult to trace the dye that causes it."

Our forebears discovered the value of leaves, barks, roots, nuts and flowers as colouring material, and over the centuries various combinations came into use. Dark women in Greece and Rome sometimes dyed their hair golden with a mixture of quince juice and privet, while the raven-haired women of Turkey created a supple, shiny, black effect on their hair with a preparation of gallnuts, first dried in oil and rubbed in salt and then added to a complicated combination of crushed pomegranate flowers, gum arabic, henna and that uniquely Turkish invention, *rastik-yuki,* which is a combination of iron and copper. Arab women, on the other hand, used just henna for auburn shades or henna and indigo to create a blue-black combination, or for simpler effect an essence made of green oranges steeped in oil for several weeks to conquer grey hair.

Many of the plant and vegetable substances which are useful for dyeing can be added to your herbal shampoo.

Henna Colouring—Brown, Auburn, Black, Red

Henna is a non-toxic dye which is not a primary sensitizer or irritant. It has been used for thousands of years in the Near and Far East. Unfortunately, henna dyeing is a long, tedious process, and it is rather difficult to stabilize the colour except with experience. The colour lasts several months, however, and with experimentation you can achieve a rich auburn, brown or black or an interesting red. Since henna is slightly astringent, be sure to rub a light covering of safflower or corn oil on your scalp before using it.

Hair must be shampooed before using henna. Wear gloves during the entire application as henna can stain hands and fingernails. (For henna nail-polish application see Chapter VII.)

henna powder	2 cups
warm water	1 cup
pure vinegar	1 teaspoon

optional

goldenseal root (powdered)	½ teaspoon

Stir henna powder and water into thick paste. Add vinegar to help release dye. Add optional golden seal. Let stand for one hour. Stir the henna, vinegar, golden seal in the top of a double boiler until the water in the bottom pot boils vigorously. Remove from flame and let stand for 1 hour. Heat up again quickly, and with gloved hands massage into hair. For a brown colour let the hair stand in a linen towel for at least 3 to 4 hours. For auburn or dark hair colour let the colour stay in up to 6 hours. Then wash the hair. Keep rinsing until the water comes away very clear. Keep combing the hair as you rinse. To counteract drying action gently massage oil into the scalp.

Other Red Hair Dyes

There are several other vegetables that will dye the hair a reddish colour. A strong infusion of radish and privet mixed together and washed through the hair will turn it red. Saffron will also give the hair a reddish tint, as will marigold flowers.

Other Black or Brown Hair Dyes

Walnut shells make another harmless dye which progressively adds colour to the hair. Before the nuts are ripe, crush the green outer shells in a mortar and cover with water. Add a touch of table salt. Let stand 3 days. Now add 3 cups of boiling water and simmer for 5 hours, always making sure the evaporated water is replaced. (Make a mark on the pot.) Express the dark liquid from the shells by means of a press or by twisting the shells in a cloth. Replace separated liquid in pot again and now reduce to a quarter of its volume. Add a dozen drops of perfume if you wish, and some fixative of alum and a touch of glycerine to soften the hair. Use on shampooed, clean hair. At first it will produce a somewhat yellowish effect, but it will finally give the hair a good deep black colour.

Other woods which can be used for dyeing the hair are catechu, logwood, brazilwood, quebracho, sandalwood and some redwood. Make a decoction of 4 tablespoons of any of these woods in a pint of water. Simmer for 20 minutes to ½ hour. Strain and brush through hair again and again. Also rinse

through hair. These are progressive dyes. Best results will be
seen after several applications.

Culpeper says "hair of the head washed with berries (elder
berries) boiled in wine is made black."

Golden Hair Dyes

Many Northern Italian women have natural golden red hair
which was immortalized by the Venetian painter Titian and the
Florentine painter Botticelli, particularly in his "Birth of Venus."
During the Venetian ascendancy as a sea power, especially during the Renaissance, this exquisite hair colour was duplicated
with dyes throughout the world. The colour was so distinctive
that there are many references to it in literature, where it is
referred to as *capelli file d'oro* (golden thread hair). Titian's
cousin, Cesare Vicallio, reported that many dark-haired Venetian
and other Italian beauties who wished to attain this colour,
spent "hours under the solana, a special crownless hat with a
huge brim which was used to spread their long hair on as they
sat on the roofs of their palazzos to dry their hair after it had
been dipped in liquid dyes."

I do not know the formula for golden thread hair, but it
was probably henna with some citric acid base.

Chamomile

This white and yellow flower lightens mousy or blond hair.
You can use it either as a rinse or as a dye. If you just want
highlights, infuse a handful of the flowers in a pint of boiling
water, steep for a few hours and strain. As with all *special rinses*
arrange to have an extra basin to catch the drippings so that
you can keep rinsing your hair until the colour is right.

For a rinse, make a strong infusion by adding 1 pint of
boiling water to 2 to 4 tablespoons of chamomile flowers. Steep
for 20 minutes to 3 hours. Strain, and rinse through hair again
and again. For a dye, make a paste of 1 cup of the infusion and
½ cup of kaolin clay. Apply paste to hair for varying periods

from 15 minutes for a lightening effect to 60 minutes for a warmer blond tint.

For extra highlights to rinse or dye add quassia chips. First simmer chips to soften them and add to chamomile while steeping to make infusion. Strain.

Rhubarb Root Golden Dye

This is by far the most effective herbal hair lightener that I have experimented with. Even the very first rinse or application results in a heavenly honey gold look, which becomes softer and deeper gold as it is applied again. If you can sit in the sun after using it, this seems to enhance the colour and strengthen the effect of the dye. Rhubarb roots can dye dark blond hair golden, or lighten brown hair to a rich golden colour. Use gloves with this dye as it can stain the palms and fingernails, although it washes off quite easily.

rhubarb root	4 tablespoons
water	1½ pints
(or white wine)	

Simmer root in water or wine for 20 minutes. Steep for several hours. Strain twice. Rinse through the hair several times or use as a paste. Paste will dye hair more effectively, especially at the roots. To make the paste, add ½ a cup of kaolin powder to a cup of decoction. (To counteract possible drying action add beaten egg yolk and ½ teaspoon of cider vinegar and a teaspoon of glycerine to condition the hair). The wine in fact works best, but is quite sticky and must be rinsed off, whereas the water infusion can be left on the hair.

Saffron Dip

Trotula, a famous ancient doctor, left the following recipe. For making the hair golden mix equal parts of elder bark, flowers of broom and saffron, plus the beaten yolk of an egg boiled in water. Skim off the pomade that floats to the surface and use as a hair dye.

Mullein

These interesting plants are common in meadows and wastelands, growing alone, with fuzzy, greenish leaves. Their leaves in an infusion, steeped, strained and rinsed through the hair, will make a golden colour.

Honey Dye

Here is another successful old-fashioned and harmless dye made of honey and gum arabic. It is more difficult to make than the ones just mentioned since it requires distilling. But if you have an old-fashioned perfume still, or have access to such a device in a home laboratory, or want to make a home still, it is worthwhile because it is effective and nourishing for the hair.

"Take the best honey, 2 pints, gum arabic, 2 ounces. Distill them with a gentle fire. The first water which comes forth doth whiten the face, the second and third make the hair yellow."

To Turn Grey Hair Dark

People have always spent a lot of time and money working out "waters" to darken the hair to its original colour. Ralph Harry points out that it is unlikely that such historical personages as Marie Antoinette or Sir Thomas More *suddenly* turned grey while in prison. "Hair washes and dyes have been known since the earliest days," writes Harry. "In the case of political and other prisoners, it is more than likely that those incarcerated no longer had access to their favourite dye. Uncharitable, but possibly a much more likely scientific explanation of any such occurrence."

Among the dyes for darkening hair and hiding the grey are infusions of leaves of the wild vine, artichoke, mulberry tree, fig tree, raspberry bush, myrtle; decoctions of roots of the holm oak and caper tree; decoction of barks of the willow, walnut tree and pomegranate; decoction of shells of beans, gall and cypress nuts; green shells of walnuts, ivy berries, cockles; red beet seeds, poppy flowers, alum. Also sage, marjoram, balm, betony, laurel infusions.

The Arabs use the essence of green oranges steeped in oil for several weeks to restore colour to greying black hair.

An old recipe says your hair will turn black if, after you have washed it, you dip your comb in oil-of-tartar and comb it through three times a day while in the sun.

Dried or fresh sage will darken grey hair. It can be added to the shampoo and also used as a rinse. Make a strong infusion of at least 4 tablespoons to a pint of boiling water, and apply the strained and steeped liquid with a sponge or cotton wool to the roots of the hair. A long-lasting sage hair-darkener can be made with a pint of dark sage tea, a pint of bay rum, and 1 ounce of glycerine. Bottle and label and apply to roots each night until hair reaches desired colour.

Tag alder root, or red alder, produces another dye which will gradually darken the hair brown. You can experiment with the amount needed but can make a weak solution with 1 ounce and a pint of boiling water. Simmer for 20 minutes, steep for several hours, strain and use with sponge or cotton wool on roots of hair. To preserve, use the same proportions of bay rum and glycerine as in the sage recipe.

CHAPTER V

EYES

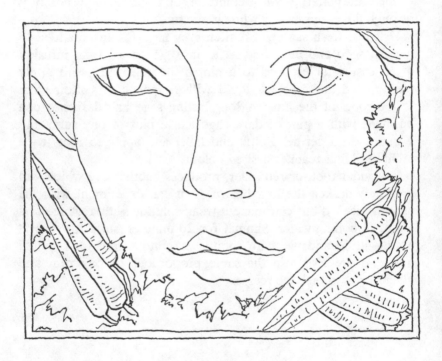

Have you ever noticed how quickly your eyes respond to negative and positive stimuli? How shiny and bright they look when
you are happy and relaxed, how dull when tired? How smog
and smoky rooms make them bloodshot, and how lack of sleep
will cause shadows and puffiness under them? The eyes are in-
timately connected with the brain and other parts of the body,

and immediately reflect unhappiness or malfunctioning—as with the yellow look from a gall bladder or liver attack, for instance.

Food and the Eyes

Though I am a supporter of many old remedies and herbal aids, it becomes more and more obvious that all these aids must be used in conjunction with cleansing and purifying foods, and foods which will regenerate the cells and revitalize your complexion, your hair and the rest of you.

In ancient Egypt doctors realized the connection between the eyes and food intake, and advised liver, which is high in vitamin A, for several diseases of the eye. Today's nutritionists know that for good eye care you have to have an adequate intake of vitamin A, C and B every day, and traces of other supplements and minerals.

The herbalist Jethro Kloss, in *Back to Eden,* says that eye troubles "are caused mainly from a deranged stomach," and that the main thing is "to eat food which will give you a pure bloodstream." He gives a long list of such cleansing herbs, and adds that fruits, fruit juices, cucumbers, carrots, celery and leafy vegetables are cleansing to the system. He advises taking the juice of a lemon in hot water 1 hour before breakfast each morning. I find that 1 tablespoon of cider vinegar in a glass of water, (with or without 1 tablespoon of honey) has a fantastic energizing and cleansing effect.

Several vegetables are very helpful for eye strain. Carrot is the most important, since it contains a large amount of vitamin A. Others are celery, parsley, chicory, spinach and escarole. I tried these when having trouble with my own eyes, when new glasses and eye exercises were not proving completely successful, and the effect was magical. Make juices with an extractor, using fresh washed vegetables, preferably not those which have been sprayed with insecticide.

29. SLEEP

A renowned nineteenth-century beauty wrote that the best recipe for bright eyes is keeping good hours: "Just enough regular and natural sleep is the great kindler of woman's most charming light." Many models have told me that they couldn't function, and their eyes would start looking crepey, if they didn't get between 8 and 10 hours' sleep a night. See Chapter IX for natural aids to sleep.

Resting During the Day

Before I discovered the vitamin deficiencies that were keeping me down, I used to long to take a nap every afternoon. Now I don't need one. But when I write most of the day I find that my shoulders, neck and eyes become very tired, and I often do relaxing eye exercises. I frequently lie down and use one of the soothing herbal eye aids, and 10 or 15 minutes later I can get up completely refreshed. It is best to lie with the feet higher than the head, as this gives the body a needed reversal in gravity and circulation. This is most refreshing to the eyes and other parts of the body.

30. EYE REFRESHERS

Cucumber

Cucumber is not only easily available but tones up the eye membranes, and cools and soothes inflamed eyes. Peel a piece of cucumber and squeeze the juice right into your eye. Or use a slice of peeled cucumber instead of an eye pad.

Witch Hazel

Witch hazel is another valuable eye aid, and can immediately reduce eye puffiness. Pour the extract over cotton-wool pads, or better still use the witch hazel ice cold.

Eyebright

My grandmother was never without a jar of strong infusion of the revered old herb eyebright in her icebox, and I follow her example by keeping some at all times in my refrigerator. I use it whenever I can. Father Kunzle, in *Herbs and Weeds*, reports that the whole herb is used to strengthen the eyes, and that the "ancients boiled it in wine and drank it at bedtime." Father Kneipp, in *My Water Cure*, also recommends it for washing the eyes.

Recently a friend came to my house after a long tiring day, and while we were dressing for the opera she asked if I had anything for the dark circles under her eyes. I mentally hovered over several remedies, but finally suggested the ice-cold eyebright—and a 15-minute rest. The circles quickly disappeared.

Chamomile, Wormwood and Other Herbs

Chamomile infusion is also a favourite eye aid and is very soothing when used as a compress.

Wormwood infusion is effective for eye inflammation, while a horsetail decoction will bring down swelling of the eyelids.

Jethro Kloss recommends 1 teaspoon of *red raspberry leaves,* 1 teaspoon of *witch hazel leaves* in a cup of boiling water for a wet eye pack. Strain to use. He also recommends fennel tea as a drink and for eye bathing (dilute the tea by a third). Also highly recommended is one of his favourite herbs—*goldenseal* mixed in equal parts of 1 teaspoon each with *boric acid* in a pint of boiling water. Shake, allow to settle and then use. Fennel, eyebright and chamomile can be used together for soothing the eyes. Use ⅛ teaspoon of each in 1 cup of boiling water, strain and cool.

In addition to the herbs mentioned previously you can also use marigolds, rosemary, teasel, celandine, sassafras, plantain, daisy, elder, linseed, lily of the valley, common marjoram and violets; and eating vegetables like endive, strawberries, parsley and potatoes can help.

31. PUFFINESS AND CIRCLES

Chronic dark circles can have many causes, such as insomnia, fatigue or strain. Grated potato applied to the swelling helps reduce it. Also experiment with chamomile, eyebright, wormwood, goldenseal infusions, or witch hazel extract.

Rose hip tea can reduce under-eye puffiness. So can the application of a fresh fig. Papaya tea or papaya mint tea can also reduce dark circles under the eyes.

Many people with exceptional chronic puffiness under the eyes will respond to a daily kidney-flushing treatment, and doctors often recommend drinking no less than 8 glasses of water a day. Since the vital mineral in potassium is often washed away in this flushing, add additional grapefruit or orange or banana to your diet. You can use nettle tea as a natural diuretic. Some bottled mineral waters will help eliminate waterlogging from the system.

32. CREAM FOR BELOW THE EYES

There is no such thing as a cream to *eliminate* wrinkles, but the following eye cream will clean the area under your eyes—a delicate area prone to dryness—and keep it lubricated and soft. The eyes are very delicate, and if you are allergy-prone you should be most careful in using any special cream around the eyes.

anhydrous lanolin (solid or liquid)	3 tablespoons
mineral oil	1 tablespoon
egg yolk	1
beeswax	2 tablespoons
safflower oil	2 tablespoons
cold water	1 tablespoon (optional)

The mineral oil is included here because it helps cleanse eye make-up from the eyes. If you like, you can use another table-spoon of melted lanolin instead.

Melt the lanolin and mineral oil together in a double boiler until the mixture gels a little. Add beaten egg yolk. In another double boiler melt beeswax and safflower oil. Add the beeswax and the safflower oil to the lanolin, mineral oil and egg yolk. Add water if you wish, as this helps moisturize, though the water sometimes gives the cream a smarting effect. Beat the mixture until frothy. Jar and label.

33. EYE EXERCISES

The Cat

The following relaxing exercise can be done at any time, but it is most effective in the early morning when your eyes are unstrained.

Get down on your stomach and lie with your head to one side, and your arms by your side, palms up. Slowly, as if you were a cat, open your eyes facing the ground and gradually look around to the side and up to the ceiling. Reverse the sequence. Shift your face to the other side and repeat the movement.

Squaring the Circle

Do not move your head during these eye movements:

Lift your eyes to the ceiling. Shift them to the floor. Repeat 10 times. Rest eyes.

Lift your eyes on a right diagonal to the ceiling and shift them to the opposite corner diagonally to the left. Repeat 10 times. Rest eyes.

Lift your eyes on a left diagonal to the ceiling and shift them to the opposite corner diagonally to the right. Repeat 10 times. Rest eyes.

Make a circle with your eyes by shifting them up on the left, round to the right, down again on the right and over to the left (clockwise). Repeat 5 times. Rest eyes.

Repeat circling anti-clockwise. Repeat 5 times. Rest eyes. Circling rate may be increased as you gain muscle control.

For a relaxing finale, rub your palms together about 6 times to cause heat and friction. Place palms gently over your eyes with fingers touching the hairline. Let your eyes absorb the full heat and darkness of the palms. When the heat evaporates, pull down the fingers so that they stroke the closed eyes several times. Stroke the fingers across the eyes towards the temples.

The following palming method seems to bring blood to the eyes and leave them feeling refreshed. With elbows supported on a table, cup a palm over each eye so that no light can enter. Open the eyes and stare into the blackness for about 2 minutes. (This method can be combined with the previous one in which you rub the palms briskly together to create heat.)

A third effective palming method, which can be alternated with the other two, relieves the tension of eye muscles and creates additional circulation of eye fluid. Close both eyes, and press the heels of your hands into your eye sockets until you gradually see "black." This can be done every 15 minutes when you are doing close work or reading.

CHAPTER VI

MOUTH AND TEETH

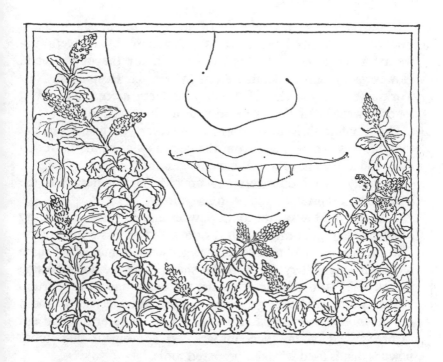

Jack London was first a sailor, then an author and still later a journalist. When he was in a little village in Korea reporting the Russo-Japanese War, the mayor came up to his hotel room to say that the entire populace was gathered in the village square to see him. Naturally London felt quite proud that his writing reputation had preceded him, but when he walked up the special platform they had erected, the mayor only asked him to take out his set of artificial teeth. For half an hour they kept him there taking out his teeth and putting them back again to the enthusiastic applause of the populace.

You don't have to take out your teeth to please the crowd, but you should be careful to preserve them.

34. BRUSHING THE TEETH

There are now two schools of thought on brushing teeth. For years, dentists have advised patients to brush teeth upward for the lower teeth, and downward for the upper teeth. However, a group of dentists from the French Hospital in New York says that you should brush your teeth *across,* and use a lot of unwaxed dental floss to rid your teeth of plaque.

Use a natural-bristle toothbrush whenever you can. Excellent toothbrushes can be made from the peeled twigs of the flowering dogwood as they have whitening effect on the teeth.

A lovely idea I discovered in an old English herbal is the coral stick. I reprint the recipe in its entirety.

"Make a stiff Paste with tooth powder and a sufficient quantity of mucilage of gum tragacanth. Form with this Paste little cylindrical rolles, the thickness of a large goose quill, and about three inches in length. Dry them in the shade. The method of using these corals, is to rub them against the teeth, and in proportion as they waste, the teeth get cleaner; they serve instead of tooth powders, opiates or prepared roots, but they are brittle and apt to break, and on this account are less convenient than tooth powder that is used with the prepared roots."

Tooth Powders

Lemon peel will take the brown stains off the teeth. Rinse the mouth thoroughly after using.

One of the oldest and most perfect tooth cleansers is common salt with water. Make a light paste and dip the brush into it.

Another favourite of mine is the strawberry. Squash a fresh strawberry in the mouth and rub against each tooth. It leaves a delightful clean taste.

Sage was used by the American Indians as a mouth cleanser and is still used today by many Arab people. Use the leaves alone or combine with a touch of honey and charcoal made from bread. As an alternative to sage you can use celandine leaves.

Several roots were once used as the base for home tooth powders. Grind equal parts of bistort root, bayberry root and prepared chalk.

Camphorated chalk has two virtues, being an inert substance and antiseptic. It is therefore valuable for dental purposes. Make a paste as follows:

camphor BP	1 teaspoon
sugar	1 lump
crushed almonds	1 tablespoon
distilled water	½ pint

Powder the camphor BP and the sugar. Grind the almonds. Mix together. Add the water and make into a paste.

35. THE MOUTH

Mouthwashes

Sunflower seeds are high in vitamin A, phosphorus, fluorine and calcium, and therefore have a marked effect on the teeth (as well as the eyes) and can help to control bleeding gum condition in a relatively short time.

Rose water can be used as an aromatic gargle and mouthwash. (There is an inexpensive recipe for rose water in Chapter X.)

The following combination of herbs makes a delightful mouthwash. Steep ¼ teaspoon of rosemary, anise and mint leaves in a pint of boiling water. Strain. Pour into labelled jar.

A Spicy Mouthwash

crushed cloves	2 tablespoons
crushed nutmeg	2 tablespoons
ground cinnamon	1 tablespoon
caraway seeds	1 tablespoon
sherry	½ pint
spirits of lavender	10 drops
(or spirits of peppermint)	

Grind all the ingredients together in a marble mortar and pour into sherry. Soak for 3 or 4 days and add either the lavender spirits or peppermint spirits. This is a highly concentrated mouthwash. Use only a few drops in a glass of water.

Small amounts of the following herbs can also be used in mouthwashes: mallow flowers, leaves of the bugle, pellitory of the wall, with honey and water.

The best mouthwash of all is probably peppermint infusion. At home we always keep a batch of fresh peppermint "tea" in the refrigerator to use as a mouthwash and a drink. It is very cleansing to the mouth, and as a drink cleanses the entire system. Apple juice, with its natural acids, is also excellent for a home mouthwash.

Many of the old herbals praise lavender water for teeth and gum care. One old recipe book describes it as follows: "Beyond doubt it is of infinite service. This simple and innocent remedy is a certain preservative, the success of which has been confirmed by long experience."

Lavender water not only makes a fine mouthwash, but can be used also in other ways. It is strongly aromatic and can be employed as a cologne, and to scent the bath. When used in a footbath, it helps cure body and foot fatigue, and a few drops on the head can alleviate a headache.

Myrrh is a resinous substance that is excellent for the mouth area since it is a mild disinfectant and a local stimulant to the mucous membranes. Myrrh can be melted down and added to any other mouthwash (it acts also as a preservative to the wash), or you can buy tincture of myrrh at the chemist's. Use a few drops at a time added to eau de cologne or water. It is reputed to be an aid in curing spongy and ulcerated gums.

Breath Sweeteners

Your mouth will feel sweet and tangy if you have a diet that is right for your system, properly eliminate waste materials, brush your teeth clear of food debris, rinse your mouth out and eat foods high in chlorophyll.

Chlorophyll, as is well known, is the green pigment found in plants. Interestingly enough, much of the commercial chlorophyll found in breath-sweetening tablets on the market is extracted from the much-used cosmetic herb, nettle. But this commercial product is treated with an alkali to change it chemically to a salt (chlorophyllin). You can get the same effect without the alkali, by chewing large amounts of chlorophyll-rich foods.

Two such foods are parsley and watercress, and they are cleansing both for your system and for your complexion. The tops of beets, turnips and radishes are also high in chlorophyll. I use them in my juice extractor and add them to beets, carrots, celery or apple drinks. If you live in the country you can try using nettle tips for their chlorophyll content.

Balsam for Chapped Lips

Take 2 tablespoons of clarified honey, add a few drops of lavender (or any aromatic water). Mix. Keep in a labelled jar and rub on your lips before you go to sleep.

CHAPTER VII

HANDS

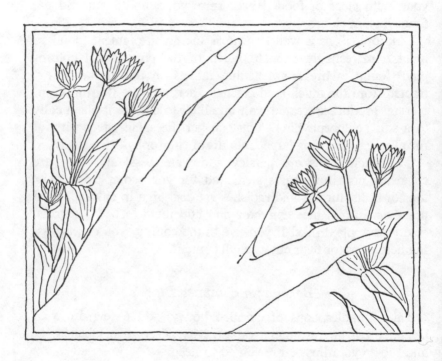

Hands are probably one of the best examples of the double standard. For while most of us respect a man with strong work-hardened hands, and accept the mechanic's or factory worker's stained hands, we expect a woman, no matter what her work, no matter what her age, to have soft, delicate and clean hands at all times. As a city dweller most of the year, a housewife, cook, gardener and full-time writer I can testify how difficult this is to achieve.

36. HAND PROTECTORS

The first antidote for dirty knuckles, dirt in nails and the cracked look which comes from repetitive chores around the house is, of course, gloves. Be sure to keep a pair under your kitchen sink, as they will help save your hands. Also replace any harsh overalkaline soaps with a glycerine or coconut-oil soap even in the kitchen. Of course this soap will not clean pots or sinks, so wear gloves when you use scouring powder or steel wool pads.

Lemon, Vinegar, Brandy

Lemon should also be a mainstay in the kitchen as it does yeoman service as a whitener, softener and nail and cuticle cleaner as well as a remedy for fishy hands, and of course it helps restore the acid coating the skin needs. If you can remember, touch the lemon to your elbows after using it on your hands and it will keep them soft and pliable too.

A charming nineteenth-century toiletry book has the following note: "If the hands are inclined to be rough and to chap, the following wash will remedy the evil: 3 ounces each of lemon juice and white wine vinegar and ½ a pint of brandy."

Ordinarily lemon tends to attract mould after a while, but the brandy and the vinegar preserve it, and each has a special use in hand care. If you prefer, you can use either the lemon or the vinegar alone.

Protective Barrier Cream

If you are doing any particularly hard manual work, make up a vegetable or nut cream protective barrier.

kaolin	1 teaspoon
(or fuller's earth)	
almond oil	1 teaspoon
egg yolk	1

Mix all three together and rub into hands and under the nails, and around the fingers and wrists. Allow to dry. At conclusion of work, wash off. This is far better for your hands than most chemically prepared protective creams on the market.

37. HAND RESTORERS

Almonds

In an old book, *A Plain Plantain,* I found the following recipe:

Take a pound of Sun Raysons; stone ym; take a pound of Bitter Almonds; blanch ym & beat ym; in stone mortar, with a glass of sack take ye peel of one Lemond, boyle it tender; take a quart of milk, & pint of Ale & make therewith a Possett; take all ye Curd & putt it to ye Almonds; yn putt in ye Rayson: Beat all these till they come to a fine Past, & putt in a pott, and keep it for ye use.

When I discover that I have been negecting my hands I use a quick version of my grandmother's hand remedy, and it never fails. I take either almond meal moistened with a little milk, or almond oil, and make a paste with a yolk of an egg, a few drops of cider vinegar, and a large spoonful of pure honey. I apply this to my hands and cover them with cotton gloves. Almond oil, by the way, is quite stable and won't go rancid if you keep it.

Glycerine and Rose Water

Glycerine and rose water are an ancient standby, and their effectiveness is explained in a modern formula book by the chemist R. G. Harry when he notes that the glycerine acts as a moisturizer by obtaining water from the lower skin layer and creating a natural moisture equilibrium.

You will find a glycerine-rose water combination at the chemist's, but since this preparation is a bit thick for my taste I often make my own version by using 4 tablespoons of glycerine to every ½ cup of my homemade rose water, which I make by adding a small vial of rose oil to a gallon of distilled water. For a thickened hand-cream version, heat 2 tablespoons of glycerine, 2 tablespoons of cornflour with ½ cup of rose water until it thickens.

Other satisfactory versions of glycerine and rose water are made by adding either a touch of lemon, or cider vinegar, or cider vinegar and honey (¼ teaspoon each).

A Spanish Pomade

You can use this or any rose water and glycerine as many times as you wish, and certainly it is safer and less taxing than the efforts made in the 1800s by certain Spanish ladies. The nineteenth-century dancer Lola Montez described their tortures as follows: "Spanish ladies take, if possible, more pains with their hands than with their faces. There is no end of the tricks to which they resort to render them delicate and beautiful. Some of the devices are not only painful, but exceedingly ridiculous. For instance, I have known some of them to sleep every night with their hands held up to the bed posts by pulleys, hoping by that means to render them pale and delicate. Both Spanish and

French women—those at least who are very particular to make the most of these charms—are in the habit of sleeping in gloves which are lined or plastered over with a pomade."

Lola Montez described the pomade as consisting of a pound of soap, a gill of salad oil, an ounce of mutton tallow boiled and mixed with a gill of spirits of wine added just before the mixture became cold.

Oatmeal

Oatmeal is another hand cleaner-restorer which can soothe rough or red skin. You can either wash with the old-fashioned oatmeal or, better still, in my opinion, since it can be used in powder form and never becomes rancid, use colloidal oatmeal. Oatmeal and water were the legendary base for the famed Countess of Jersey's beauty, and she is said to have used a fresh preparation of oatmeal on her hands, face, neck and shoulders each morning to preserve her beauty to old age.

In many parts of England they still use oatmeal and water plus a few drops of simple tincture of benzoin plus a teaspoon of almond meal as a whitening hand cleaner. For especially chapped hands a nineteenth-century ladies' manual advised bathing the hands in a mixture of linseed oil and bitter almond oil, and afterwards rinsing in a water to which simple tincture of benzoin is added.

Cocoa Butter

Cocoa butter is an effective skin softener for the hands. Equal parts of cocoa butter, oil of sweet almonds and white wax (preferably beeswax) can be melted together, stirred until cool and kept in a labelled, dark glass jar.

Cucumber

Cucumber added to the gelling irish moss (or carragheen) and gum tragacanth, glycerine and a preservative such as alcohol make up a fresh-smelling, long-lasting hand cream.

gum tragacanth	1 teaspoon
irish moss	1 teaspoon
boric acid	1 teaspoon
borax	1 teaspoon
glycerine	2 ounces
ethyl alcohol (70%)	3 ounces
peeled cucumber	

Add a touch of really hot water, enough to mix the gum tragacanth and irish moss until they dissolve. Add boric acid and borax. When all of these have been completely dissolved add the glycerine and ethyl alcohol and finally the whole cucumber. Blend. Put this into a 16-ounce bottle, add enough hot water to fill the bottle and add a few drops of perfume to your own personal taste.

Hand Care Herbs

An infusion of any of the following used as a compress is excellent for chapped or roughened hands: fennel, yarrow, marigold petals, lady's mantle, chamomile, comfrey or mallow.

38. RECONDITIONING THE NAILS

The visible nail is hard plate and made out of protein and smaller amounts of calcium, phosphorus and trace metals. It grows fastest in youth and slows down later. The nails are like the eyes, hair, and skin in indicating general and specific health. Have you ever noticed how carefully a doctor looks at your nails when he is giving you a thorough examination? Lack of colour, split or soft nails, white spots and cross or longitudinal lines, even dents, are indications and "medical history" to the trained eye.

The following cautionary programme should be followed:

Use gloves for housework.
Use barrier creams on hands and under nails for manual work.
Avoid contact with any harsh chemicals and detergents.
Dial with a metal dialer or a pencil.
File nails round, not pointed.
Avoid drying nail lacquer or remover.
Don't use plastic press-on nails.

Diet to Help Nails

Increased vitamin A for nail growth.
Increased vitamin B complex and vitamin D to cure deficiencies indicated by ridges.
Calcium tablets.
Brewer's yeast to cure hangnails and split nails (also complete source of B complex).
Colourless gelatine. Although this is an *incomplete* protein it does help many nail problems.
Horsetail tea every night to help in regeneration of nails.
A tablespoon of cider vinegar in a glass of water before meals to increase strength of nails.

On-the-nail Reconditioning

Use only a wooden stick to clean under the nails.
File with a large diamond-cut metal file or large emery board.
Increase circulation on nail by buffing. Beeswax is excellent for this.
To overcome extreme drying of nails from nail enamel, if you use it, add castor oil to the *acetone* nail polish remover.

39. NAIL AIDS AND POLISH

Cuticle Softener

Combine 2 tablespoons of fresh pineapple juice from raw pineapple (in juicer), or papaya juice, with 2 tablespoons of egg yolk and ½ teaspoon of cider vinegar. Soak nails for ½ hour. Pineapple and papaya contain an enzyme which can soften protein tissue.

Nail Restoration Cream

Combine equal parts of honey, avocado oil and egg yolk plus a pinch of sea salt. Rub into nails. Allow to remain for ½ hour. Rinse off.

Nail Strengtheners

A 5-minute soak in warm olive oil, or in a horsetail infusion, or in cider vinegar. Lemon peel rubbed on fingernails strengthens and also cleans and whitens.

Henna Nail Polish

Make a thin paste by adding warm water to henna powder. Apply to nails with a small paintbrush. Allow to dry, preferably in the sun. When thoroughly dry, rinse off in tepid water. This will give you a soft amber pink which will not chip.

CHAPTER VIII

FEET

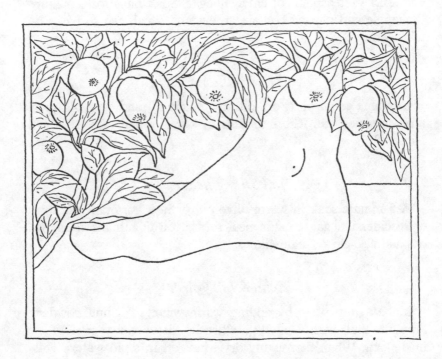

Some time ago the eminent scientist Dr. Harlow Shapley described what he assumed people from another universe might look like *if* they existed. After supplying them with various bodily mechanisms similar to, but not exactly the same as, our own, he conjectured that they would walk not on two, but on *four* legs. Dr. Shapley seemed to think this made more sense. The prevalence of back and foot problems indicates that man was not really made to stand erect on two feet. And those of us who do stand a lot each day long for respite. Learn to pamper your feet with exercise designed to eliminate accumulated toxins and to increase circulation. Experiment with hand massage, and as many stimulating and reviving foot baths and anti-fatigue herbs as you possibly can.

40. EXERCISES

You should never get out of bed without first stretching your limbs and body like a cat. Arch your ankles, bend your toes, flex your entire leg forward, back, sideways and manipulate the toes, heel and ankle forward and back. Whenever you have the chance massage your feet.

Draining Away Fatigue

Getting off your feet after an extremely hard day is a good idea, and it helps if you don't merely lie down, but attempt to drain away the accumulated toxins by lying with your feet higher than your head, and gently massaging the legs, one at a time, from the foot to the knee. This helps the circulation and practically pushes the toxins out of your legs. For a 10-minute relaxing exercise, see page 101.

Weak Feet Exercises

There are many simple exercises which will help you to strengthen your feet:

Flex and rotate your ankles.
Flex and rotate each toe by hand.
Rise slowly on your toes and go down again. Repeat several times.
Walk barefoot in the sand, mud or grass.
Pick up marbles with your toes.
Walk first on the outside and then the inside of each foot.

Do as much swimming as you can.

Walk, kick, lift, fold, knead and massage your legs and feet under water.

Foot baths of willow bark are suggested by Father Kunzle for convalescents or the old.

Foot baths of hay flowers are suggested by Father Kneipp, and of bed straw by Culpeper.

41. HERBS AND BATHS AGAINST FATIGUE

Elderberry

My grandmother wore crushed elderberry leaves in her shoes when she felt tired or wished to prevent fatigue. She reduced the leaves to a fine powder in her mortar and usually added a small amount of fuller's earth, to make it into a kind of talcum powder.

Fern

Father Kunzle writes that "people who take long walks will lose every tiredness if they stuff fern leaves in their shoes and fill their pockets with it." Ferns can be found in profusion by the wayside, and also in every florist's shop.

Hot-cold Foot Bath

Shocking the feet with alternate hot, cold, hot, cold foot baths (ending with cold) will often help eliminate foot fatigue.

Hay Flower Foot Bath

Father Kneipp describes hay flower foot baths as being extremely efficacious for all ailments of the feet including corns, ingrowing toe nails, walking blisters, sweating feet, problem feet of all kinds. He recommends using 5 handfuls of the hay flowers, with stalks, leaves, blossoms, seed, even the hay itself, to a quart of boiling water, and soaking your feet in the tepid mixture. He also mentions oat straw foot baths for corns and other growths. These herbs are available by post from herb sources.

Lavender

A few drops of lavender oil in a tepid foot bath will relieve fatigue immediately.

Lemon or Cider Vinegar Bath or Rub

Lemon juice softens and relieves tired feet, and a foot bath in cider vinegar can also restore vigour to your feet, as well as other parts of the body. The vinegar will also eliminate itchiness and athlete's foot.

42. FOOT AND LEG PROBLEMS

Corns and Calluses

Corns and calluses are caused by the way we walk and by friction on the foot. You are therefore better off walking barefoot or with a minimum sandal whenever possible. However, since most of us cannot do this, massaging with olive, castor oil or lanolin, or any favourite face cream, will soften the dead tissues and make it easier to rid yourself of these impediments.

Rather than the hay flower baths favoured by Father Kneipp, some people prefer yarrow and salt foot baths followed by a massage with lemon peel oil. You can make this by turning half a lemon inside out and steeping your favourite oil in the half overnight.

Another old herbal source mentions that "the juice of houseleek takes away corns from the toe and feet if they be bathed therewith every day, and at night emplastered as it were with the skin of the same houseleek." It has very healing powers for the complexion, too.

All the root bulbs have drawing power, and garlic or onion tied to corns can ease the pain. Many ancient herbal books mention roasted clove of garlic or onion used several nights in a row as a cure for corns.

Rubbing a pumice stone over calluses softened by bathing will keep calluses small and eventually eliminate them.

Leg Cramps

Father Kunzle suggests a foot bath of boiled water and wood mosses, the kind which can be found along the path in damp woods. Other herbalists recommend cranberry bark, or cramp bark, as it is sometimes called, for quick relief from leg cramps. The herbalists Wood and Ruddock say that people with leg cramps should drink cranberry bark tea night and morning for at least 14 days and "their troubles will seldom return."

According to Adelle Davis, increased vitamin C given to a test group of soldiers lessened their fatigue and leg cramps; and many dancers I know find that large doses of vitamin C and calcium tablets will control and eventually eliminate their leg cramps. Calcium tablets are also helpful in stopping the leg cramps associated with menstruation and menopause.

Varicose Veins

Father Kneipp suggests that people with varicose veins should never take baths over 88° F., or foot baths beyond the ankle area. For this complaint, you should always consult your doctor.

Fallen Arches

Fallen arches can be extremely painful and often prevent people from leading an active life. Lucas describes how a liniment of 1 ounce of powdered wormwood, steeped for a week in a pint of rum and then strained and bottled, was rubbed nightly on painful fallen arches and helped one invalid patient return to his work within three weeks. Wormwood is an aromatic herb esteemed by the Greeks as an aid to digestion and appetite, and as an expeller of worms (hence the name). It has a fine reputation as a poultice for all kinds of swelling, sprains and rheumatism.

Another liniment that is extremely useful is a blend of 2 ounces of gum myrrh, 1 ounce of goldenseal and ½ ounce of cayenne pepper in 1 quart of rubbing alcohol or a pint of cider vinegar and a pint of water.

Itching Feet

Lemon juice and cider vinegar have been mentioned before; and another food—onion—was considered excellent for controlling itching. The ancients used onion juice between the toes to relieve itching and athlete's foot. Red clover blossoms were also used by country people for this purpose. They boiled them in a small amount of water, strained it off and placed the blossoms in a cotton poultice.

Swollen Feet

Father Kunzle has these reassuring words for those whose feet swell in summer. "Do not be frightened, because it is not dangerous, even though painful. The swelling will soon disappear if you tie crushed red robin (wild geranium) over the ailing spots. At the same time drink tea plentifully made of lady's mantle, or mallow, or of the leaves and blossoms of the bindweed." The leaves of the house geranium are as efficacious as red robin.

Foot Powder

If you use a natural powder after the bath you will have less friction when you put on your shoes. The following powder is particularly effective in hot weather:

talcum powder	½ cup
powdered boric acid	2 tablespoons
cornstarch	½ cup
peppermint extract	½ teaspoon
rubbing alcohol	1 teaspoon

Mix the ingredients together into lidded labelled jar.

Perspiration of the Feet

Father Kunzle calls this "the healthiest illness in existence. It ought never to be quite suppressed because severe and incurable diseases will follow, and will last until the feet perspire again. . . . You can minimize the perspiration, but, never, never by cold foot baths, only by the cleansing of the kidneys, drinking tea of herbs which act as a strong diuretic: lady's mantle, Indian corn's beard, couch or quick grass."

Cold Feet

A little cayenne pepper in your stockings will bring you an immediate sense of warmth. To make up in advance as an outdoor talcum powder, add some inert substance such as fuller's earth, or some talcum powder.

CHAPTER IX

SLEEP

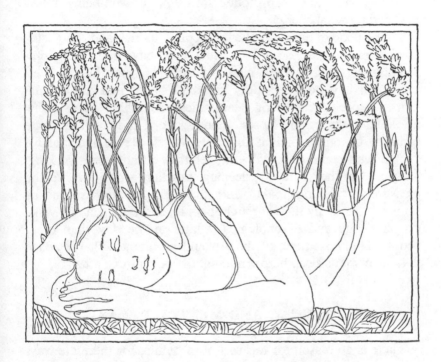

"I often think this insomnia business is about 90 per cent nonsense," said Stephen Leacock. "When I was a young man living in a boarding house in Toronto, my brother George came to visit me, and since there was no spare room, we had to share my bed. In the morning, after daylight, I said to George, 'Did you get much sleep?' 'Not a damn minute,' said he. 'Neither did I,' I rejoined. 'I could hear every sound all night.' Then we put our heads up from the bedclothes and saw that the bed was covered with plaster. The ceiling had fallen on us in the night, but we hadn't noticed it. We had 'insomnia.'"

Leacock was one of the many people who only think they don't sleep; but for people who actually toss and turn the whole night through, there are true physical manifestations. The skin on the face feels saggy and heavy, and lacks tone. Their eyes are bleary and baggy, and their entire body feels dull. On the other hand a good night's sleep produces a feeling of well-being, freshness and physical energy.

Many people have excellent sleeping habits and only stay awake on the rare occasions when they have something profoundly worrying on their mind, or have eaten too late or overeaten. Anxiety, cold feet, poor breathing habits and bad circulation are specific causes of sleeplessness. I number quite a few insomniacs among my closest friends, and if they have a single common denominator it is that they are all clever and creative people who cannot, or will not, let their minds stop working. They all say they hate not sleeping, but they won't give up the pleasures of staying up late into the night talking, reading or thinking. Basically they are night people, and they actually wake up physically and psychologically later in the day than other people. I suppose none of them would go along with the adage that "one hour's sleep before midnight is worth three after."

43. PHYSICAL AND MENTAL RELAXERS

There is no reason for this sort of insomnia, for there are ways to retrain the too active mind. Before going to bed, do a little bit of exercise—some stretching at least; get into a full warm tub, or for a real surprise, a cold foot bath, or sitz bath; and pop into bed *without drying*. Take any one of the nightcap herbal teas in the next section, and start breathing deeply. Deep breathing or deep yawning will make your body feel heavy and languid.

Breathe deeply 3 or 4 times and then hold in the last breath as long as you possibly can, and repeat this action several times.

Then, as your body and mind begin to feel drowsy, and a touch of autosuggestion. Lie down on your back; slowly and precisely concentrate on your feet, and say to yourself, "My feet are heavy, they feel heavy." Slowly think of each part of your body in the same way. Your legs are heavy, your thighs are heavy, your stomach, your chest, your arms are heavy, heavy, heavy. You feel as if you are floating on water, but now your body is too heavy for you even to lift your arms, your fingers, your wrists. Then mentally make your neck heavy—and then your lips, your nose, your eyes, your head. If you have thoroughly concentrated (and learning this intense concentration sometimes takes a little time), you can fall asleep immediately. But if you find that you are even slightly awake, lie in a comfortable position, preferably with your entire body serenely relaxed, and lift your right foot. Tense it and relax it suddenly. Do the same with your left foot. Lift your right hand. Clench it. Drop it suddenly. Do the same with your left hand. Now tighten your face in a grimace—make an ugly face. Relax it. Give in to the heaviness of your body, if necessary making each part of your body heavy again.

If you are still resisting—and it *is* a matter of resisting—try mentally writing the number 3—*slowly*. Do this as slowly as you can 3 times, and you should be fast asleep seconds later.

Relaxing Baths

Since relaxed sleep is one of the keys to good health and good looks, all the great herbalist-healers are preoccupied with sleeping aids. Father Kneipp tells of his successful water cures.

Take a cold, 1-to-3-minute foot bath with water up to the calves. According to Father Kneipp, this will "cure fatigue and produce sound and wholesome sleep."

Another suggested bath is the cold 3-to-5-minute semi-bath, either kneeling in the water so that the thighs are covered, or sitting in cold water which reaches to the pit of the stomach. Father Kneipp claims that these last two semi-baths are valuable and useful in that they have a great effect on the digestion and intestines. "It serves to regulate circulation, expel unhealthy gases, and make the body impervious to catching colds." These two baths will not only help you to fall asleep, but can be taken to advantage after a bad night's rest.

Father Kneipp insists that the body should *not* be dried with a towel. Just get straight into a warm bed and dry in your night clothes, or if the idea of that upsets you, jump into bed with a lot of towels wrapped round you. If bathing in the early morning, put your clothes on straight away and exercise until your body temperature returns to normal.

44. AIDS TO SLEEP

Foods

Calcium and vitamin D are nature's most readily available nightcaps. Warm a glass of whole or skim milk and add a tablespoon of honey and you have an old-fashioned sleeping potion. The calcium tranquillizes and the honey helps the body to retain fluids, thus keeping the kidneys from alerting you during the night. Honey can be used in any herbal tea. Nutritionists also suggest taking 2 tablets of calcium. Personally, I like calcium with magnesium.

Herbs

Most of the following herbs can be used as nightcap teas. Add 1 teaspoon to a glass of boiling water, steep and strain. Add honey if you like, particularly if getting up frequently to pass water is a problem. Most tea herbs can be extracted with 15 minutes of steeping, but if the time is longer it will be noted.

The most effective herb sleep-producer in my view is *valerian*, from the Latin *valere*, "to be in health"; it was known to the Greeks as a nerve calmer. There are no bad aftereffects from the use of this herb. It was prescribed to relieve strain brought on by the air raids in the Second World War, and even single doses proved helpful, as it quiets the nervous system and the brain.

Valerian grows in profusion in Derbyshire, and is also cultivated for world-wide sale. Unfortunately it has a bad smell. It comes in coated capsules from many herbal pharmacies, however, and can be used alone or with other sleep-producing herbs, either in capsule or tea form.

Peppermint tea is a delicate and aromatic bedtime drink, and can also be used, as can chamomile, or lime flowers (linden) for babies' sleep and teething problems. Chamomile tea is a traditional tranquillizer and linden or lime (known by its Latin name as *Tilia*) is another effective soothing tea. Even today French mothers give *Tilia* to a crying child, especially at bed-time. Honey from lime flowers is highly regarded for its flavour, and is used in many medicines and liqueurs. Prolonged bathing in lime flower infusion is a folk remedy to calm hysteria. Make sure that you have a good supplier for lime-flower tea, as flowers that are too old can produce symptoms of narcotic intoxication. For an old, effective teething remedy combine a tablespoon of peppermint, skullcap and pennyroyal in a pint of boiling water. Steep for 30 minutes, strain and use warm, with honey for sweetening, 1 teaspoon at a time.

Aromatic woodruff can greatly improve, and even prolong, one's sleep. To make the tea, use only hot, not boiling, water. According to the English herbalist Gerard, pouring woodruff into wine will "make men merry."

A hot mull which will put you to sleep is warm wine plus a few cloves, a stick of cinnamon and a touch of woodruff. Another sleep-producing drink is a toddy with warmed rum, and 6 cloves, 6 coriander seeds, 1 stick of cinnamon, a tablespoon of honey, the yolks of 2 eggs, juice of ½ lemon and a touch of woodruff.

Wild lettuce is narcotic, and all lettuce possesses some of this narcotic juice—not enough to make you drugged, of course. But the ancients held lettuce in high esteem for its cooling and re-freshing qualities. In fact the Emperor Augustus attributed his recovery from a dangerous illness to lettuce, and built an altar and erected a statue in its honour. Eau de laitre is water distilled from lettuce, and is used in France as a mild sedative in doses of 2 to 4 ounces. Certainly if you have an urge to eat something before you go to bed, try slowly chewing lettuce leaves, although the teas I have mentioned, plus honey, would be more effective.

Sage is yet another favourite sleep-producer, and a cup of sage tea plus honey will bring on a sense of calm. We always had several "sleep jars" in the house when I was a child, and one jar always contained a teaspoon of sage and rosemary to every 2 tablespoons of peppermint. Use only 1 teaspoon of the combined herbs for your steeped, strained tea before going to sleep.

The early American settlers used both *red bergamot tea* and *pennyroyal tea* for relaxed sleep. But a herb that does double duty in relaxing and picking up is *lemon balm.* It doesn't put you to sleep but rather removes any spasms and tensions which prevent sleep; and it can also be used as an early morning tea to overcome a feeling of tiredness.

Father Kunzle has two suggestions for harmless sleeping potions. He recommends 4 parts of golden rod to 1 part juniper, or a calming tea of lady's mantle and cowslips combined. Cowslips (*Primula veris*) have been used for centuries in England for nightly tea. Use flowers or root—preferably flowers.

The American herbalist Jethro Kloss advises a warm bath and hot tea for immediate sleep, and he suggests any of the following herbs steeped in a cup of boiling water for 20 minutes: lady's slipper, valerian, catnip, skullcap or hops, especially hops. He says that these herbs will not only induce sleep but will tone up the stomach and nerves, and never leave any bad aftereffect. If none of these herbs is available, hot lemonade, or hot grapefruit juice, either with or without honey, is an excellent substitute.

The Germans use ground anise with honey in warm milk as their bedtime drink, and the Dutch use another version, a tablet of aniseed in a glass of hot milk. Many Indians, I am told, use nutmeg oil on the forehead to induce sleep. The volatile *oil* does contain an intoxicant principle, but even grated nutmeg with lemon and boiling water can sometimes be used as a nightcap.

Many botanical sources and herb pharmacies have their own

combinations for sleep. They are frequently made up in the form of capsules.

Dr. Jarvis, author of *Folk Medicine*, prefers apple, grape and cranberry juice to citrus juices. Since a great deal of nightly and other unease is due to an overalkaline reaction of the blood, these juices will undoubtedly help. Dr. Jarvis also suggests a daily drink of 2 teaspoons of cider vinegar in a glass of water before breakfast each morning. If you find this difficult to take, try a tablespoon of the cider vinegar and a tablespoon of honey (preferably uncooked honey) to a glass of water, which reconstitutes to a rather apple-juice taste. It is marvellous for getting the body started in the morning, and is an effective cure for constipation—another problem which can affect sleep.

45. HERB PILLOWS

Did your grandmother have a sleep pillow—a tiny, slender herb cushion covered with muslin and gay fabric? These are particularly good for invalids, babies and anyone in need of extra help in sleeping. They are a lovely present for anyone bedridden or old. The gentle aroma emanating from the pillows soothes the nerves, and often helps overcome the sickroom smell.

My favourite of all is lavender, or lavender with crushed rosebuds, or equal parts of sage, peppermint and lemon balm with or without lavender. Add some powdered orrisroot to "fix" the aroma, or a drop of simple or compound tincture of benzoin, when you crush the herbs in the mortar. You can also add a pinch of any of the following: rosemary, lemon verbena (a heavenly clean smell), angelica, tarragon, woodruff, marjoram, dill, thyme, hops.

You can make an entire pillow of hops, or of woodruff, or indeed of any of the herbs mentioned before as herb teas. Crush the dried leaves a bit, add a fixative (see page 160), enclose in two men's handerchief's, and add a washable "pillowcase" covering of a patterned fabric. These should be quite flat and slender to be comfortable. In order not to lose them every time you change your pillowcase, attach with a safety pin to the pillow ticking.

CHAPTER X

PERFUMES

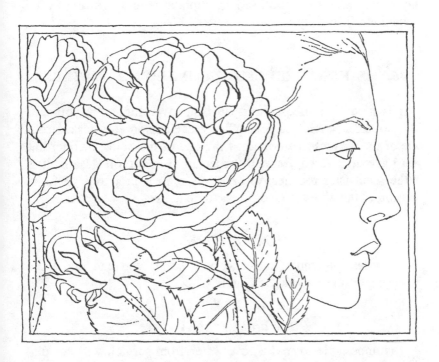

The very best perfumes are blends of several dozen ingredients. These famous perfumes are very expensive, for it takes thousands of flowers to make the best perfume essences. Modern scientific methods are so effective that any woman today can possess scents and perfumes unattainable by the greatest kings and queens of history.

However, it is still possible to obtain or make delightful spicy or floral scents without spending too much money. One way is to buy oils to use as perfume bases or on their own; another is to create your own herbal scents. Most perfumes and colognes require distilling, and whereas many homes possessed stills in the past, they are now frowned upon by the Customs and Excise (since whisky needs distilling). I have therefore concentrated on some old spicy scents that *don't* require distilling—details for potpourri recipes, aromatic waters which have several uses and scent balls which can be used in cupboards and drawers or be shaped into jewellery.

46. MAKING PERFUMES AND FLORAL WATERS

It is great fun mixing and devising a perfume for yourself. Modern science and the post office make this an easy task. From one of the sources mentioned at the end of the book, or one that you have discovered yourself, order an aromatic oil. Use as it is if the scent isn't too heavy, or dilute it in a prepared perfume solvent, obtainable from some perfume houses.

Floral Waters

For a less pungent (and cheaper) scent, you can make the following floral or aromatic waters.

Rose and Orange Water

It is impossible to make rose water from scratch without distilling, but nevertheless my favourite rose water is one I make myself, and requires only the mixing together of a gallon of distilled water and 1 ounce of essence of roses. This costs so little that I am quite liberal in my use of such rose water in my bath, or when I want to make an aromatic vinegar, or for various creams, lotions and even shampoos.

Mix the water and essence and let it age for a week or more. The longer the better. You can purchase rose (and other flower) essence from the botanical and pharmaceutical sources given at the end of the book.

Orange water is made in the same way as rose water.

Lavender Water

In addition to being a complexion water and an old remedy for headaches and fevers, lavender water is a revered scent. It can be eaten on a lump of sugar to allay nervousness or depression. The very best commercial lavender water on the market is Hopkinson's, developed over two hundred and fifty years ago.

Here are three recipes for lavender water that you can make yourself.

Fragrant Lavender Water

The following is a quick way to give a lavender aroma to water; but it eventually goes bad because of the sugar, so don't make too much of it. Put a lump of sugar and 3 drops of oil of lavender, or oil of spike, into a pint of clear distilled water, and shake. Use a glass with a narrow neck. After a week or two the water should be usable.

Lavender Tonic

This tonic can be used for the face and for headaches, fevers, nervousness and depression. Grind together in a marble mortar the following ingredients:

dried lavender flowers	2 tablespoons
cinnamon	2 tablespoons
ethyl alcohol	1 pint

optional

sweet cicely leaves, or another aromatic flower	1 tablespoon

Steep for 2 weeks in alcohol. Strain and use.

American Lavender Water

benzoic acid	1 drachm
oil of patchouli	½ drachm*
oil of lavender flowers	½ ounce
oil of cloves	15 drops
oil of wintergreen	15 drops
oil of bay leaves	½ drachm
oil of ylang ylang	10 drops
orange flower water	1 ounce
best grade of ethyl alcohol	

Dissolve the benzoic acid and the oils in the alcohol. Add the orange flower water: shake together well and let stand for 5 days. Filter through a cloth. Label the bottle. Let it stand and age for a few weeks.

47. OLD SCENTS

A Powdered Flower Perfume Base

This can be used as a base for other perfumes, or as a base for talcum powder mixed with cornflour, or alone.

Pound oak moss (lichen) and soak it in distilled or spring water for 5 days. Press out all the liquid. Moisten once again with a combination of rose water and orange water. Keep on soaking the moss until it has fully absorbed the aroma of the roses and the oranges. Press out the liquid. Pulverize the moss and add to any potpourri, perfume or scent ball, or talcum.

* A drachm is an eighth of an ounce; about a teaspoonful. So ½ drachm is a very small amount.

An Ancient Spice "Perfume"

Actually this isn't a perfume, but they called it that several centuries ago. It has a very spicy smell which many men like:

rose water	2 cups
bruised cloves	½ ounce
bay leaves	2–3
wine vinegar	2 cups

Combine rose water, cloves, chopped bay leaves and vinegar, and boil. As it reduces, add plain water to bring it to original amount. Put aside in a labelled jar for several weeks or more.

Walnut Leaves and Rose Water

Young fresh walnut leaves and rose water were considered an ideal combination for a man's scent several centuries ago. Heat ½ cup rose water and pour over 2 tablespoons walnut leaves. Steep for 3 hours.

48. POTPOURRI, SCENT BALLS AND PASTILLES

Potpourri is a blending of several dried aromatic flowers or herbs. It can be used to scent a room, drawers or a cupboard, either in a bowl or sewn into sachet bags. You can also scent your writing paper with your favourite potpourri.

General Recipe for Potpourri

There are as many recipes for potpourri as there are people who have made them. They depend to a great extent on the fresh or dried flowers you have on hand, and several elementary steps.

In general, rose leaves or lavender leaves should predominate, but don't let tradition confine you. This mixture of scented flowers, aromatic oils and fixative resins and seeds should depend on your personal preference.

If you are a gardener, gather your flowers after the dew has disappeared, and dry the flowers and leaves in the sun until evening.

The key to long life for a potpourri is in the mixture of bay salt and powdered orrisroot (which is a fine fixative for aromas). Use twice as much bay salt as orris.

Prepare the potpourri in layers: one layer of rosebuds, a layer of orris and bay salt, other layers of flowers, leaves and seeds, rose again, salt and orris again and so on until you come to the top of your jar. Close the lid and put the jar aside in a cupboard for about a month. Then gently mix the ingredients with a wooden spoon and—using either rose or other aromatic oil, or rose water—pour over enough to moisten all the layers completely.

Potpourri Suggestions

Your potpourri does not have to include all these items. Use this list as a guide for developing your own potpourri recipes. When in doubt as to combinations, use rosebuds, small amounts of cloves, nutmeg and cinnamon, and fixatives like gum benzoin, tonquin beans, and some sandalwood, and orrisroot and bay salt as in the general recipe.

For experimental purposes use some or all of the following to *predominate:*

Roses of all colours and shapes, orange blossoms, lavender flowers, lemon blossoms, lilies of the valley, pinks, lilacs, violets, narcissi, heliotrope, jonquils, sweet myrtle leaves, red carnations, jasmine, red bergamot (bee balm), costmary, leaves and flowers of meadowsweet (the favourite room-scenting herb of Queen Elizabeth I), rosemary, woodruff leaves, mint.

Smaller amounts of any of the following: bruised cloves, cinnamon, nutmeg (use two), thyme, sweet marjoram, sage and bay leaves.

Still smaller amounts of the following: yellow sandalwood, calamus root, cassia buds, gum benzoin, storax, tonquin beans.

Scent Balls and Scent Pastilles

Scent balls or scent pastilles are dried aromatic flowers and herbs melted together with a gum resin which will harden the mixture. Gums are also fixatives for aromas and will therefore help the aroma to last. They can be made in any size from small-bead size to large-ball size or disks of any size. These will harden so that they can be turned and polished on a lathe and will retain their scent for a very, very long time. If you want to make beads, pierce them with a needle while still quite soft. These scent balls can be used to scent handbags, drawers or cupboards, or in larger sizes can be sculpted into jewellery or belt buckles.

Scent Balls

To make a scent ball you use any group of potpourri ingredients (or use the recipe which follows) and pound them in a marble mortar together with some *gum tragacanth* (the ribbon variety is preferred) and rose water. The gum must be moistened a little with rose water for the whole potpourri to become sticky and dough-like. You can now form this "dough" into any shape you like.

Scent Pastille

powdered orrisroot	3 ounces
cassia	1 ounce
lavender flowers	1 ounce
cloves	1 ounce
rhodium wood	½ ounce
vanilla	1 teaspoon†
ambergris, musk,	6 grains each
attar of roses	
oil of verbena	15–20 drops
mucilage of gum tragacanth	enough to mix

I have made many variations of these scent balls with odds and ends of different flowers, seeds, gums and leaves, and they have all been successful. Be sure to let them dry in the air. Don't enclose them in plastic, as plastic covering keeps them soft and eventually allows a slight mould to form.

Queen Elizabeth's Perfume

I have included this here as it lends itself particularly to use as a scent ball. It was discovered in an undated manuscript, which said, "This perfume is very sweet and good for the time." It *doesn't* last as a perfume, but with the addition of gum tragacanth (as in the directions above for scent balls) it will last for many years. Like the scent ball it can also be made into any shape you like.

sugar	2 lumps
rose water	8 tablespoons
sweet marjoram	½ ounce
gum benzoin	2 pieces
(or tincture of benzoin	1 teaspoon)

† You can substitute 6 drops of tincture of benzoin, 6 drops of artificial ambergris and a teaspoon of rose essence or rose oil or even ½ cup rose water.

In a double boiler, crush sugar into rose water and heat. Bring to boil. Add marjoram and crushed benzoin or use tincture of benzoin. Melt and blend the ingredients together. As soon as you can comfortably handle the materials, form into desired shapes.

See Chapter XII, *Sources*, for stockists of perfumes, flower oils and waters, and ingredients for potpourri.

CHAPTER XI

COLLECTING AND DRYING HERBS

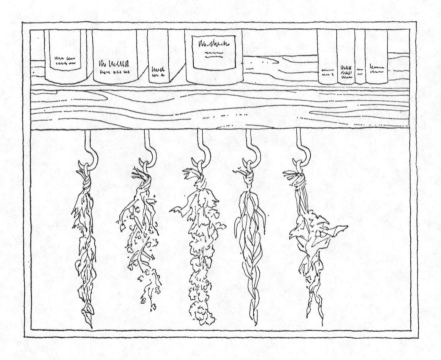

If you live in the country, you will certainly want to investigate the many weeds, wild flowers, roots and barks that you can discover either in your own garden, or by the roadside, or in wastelands or meadows. Before you use these herbs, though, on your body or hair, check whether there has been any spraying in that area. Remember, also, that by digging up a root you are destroying a wild plant—it may be better to get commercially grown roots from a herbal supplier.

Elizabeth Hall, the senior librarian of the Horticultural Society of New York, suggests the following four books as basic references in learning about herbs and weeds:

Herbs: Their Culture and Uses, Rosetta Clarkson. Macmillan.

Weeds, Dorothy Charles Hogner. Thomas Y. Crowell.

Weeds of Lawn and Garden, John M. Fogg, Jr. S-H Service Agency, Riverside, New Jersey 08075.

Wildflowers of North Eastern and North Central North America, Roger T. Peterson and Margaret McKenny. Houghton-Mifflin.

(This last book is organized by colour and is therefore helpful in identifying completely unknown plants.)

49. RULES FOR COLLECTING HERBS

Never collect herbs when they are wet, as the slightest dew, snow or frost will make the plant mouldy.

Use only perfect, unfaded, unblemished, insect-free leaves or flowers. Discard all others, as well as any thick wood stems, since they have no value. Use only unblemished roots or bark.

Gather the plant when it is in full bloom, the seed when it is ripening, the bark when it is rising. Dig roots in spring or late autumn and collect barks in spring or autumn.

50. RULES FOR DRYING HERBS

Many country people collect their herbs when they are already dried on the plant. This lessens the strength and medicinal value of herb, although it can still be used.

Scentless herbs can be dried in the sun, but herbs with an aroma should be entirely dried in the shade, after which they can be put in the sun for a short time to prevent fungus formation. Sometimes, in a cold climate, it is necessary to use heat because of the possibility of mildew. Use only slow heat.

Roots should be dried in the shade. Slice or put in bunches and store in a cool, dry, airy place.

Barks can be dried in sunlight, except wild cherry bark.

Leaves and flowers should be dried in an airy, dry place, either hung up in medium-sized bunches, or on wire mesh frames; or on shelves or tables under white shelving paper, in which case they should be turned frequently.

C. CHART: DRYING AND STORING HERBS

	Whole Plant	Bark	Flowers	Leaves	Roots
In sun	Can be picked after drying — American Indians and gypsies did this, but it lessened strength of herb.	Dry in sun. Except wild cherry bark.	Best to dry in airy dry place out of sun except for short time. Sun depletes strength of herb. No scented flowers can be dried in sun.	Best to dry in airy dry place out of sun except for short time. Although sun lessens strength of herb, unscented leaves can be dried in the sun.	
In shade			Flowers with aroma must be dried in the shade. Place in sun for short time to prevent fungus.	Leaves with aroma must be dried in shade. Put in sun for short time to prevent fungus.	Dry roots in shade.
Extra heat			Sometimes in cold climate it is necessary to use extra heat because of possibility of mildew. Use *slow* gas or electric heat only.		
Storage			Dry in medium bunches and hang in dry air, or place on wire mesh frames, or under white shelving paper, or on long tables and turn often.	Dry in medium bunches and hang in dry air, or place on wire mesh frames, or under white shelving paper, or on long tables and turn often.	Store in cool dry airy place.

CHAPTER XII

SOURCES

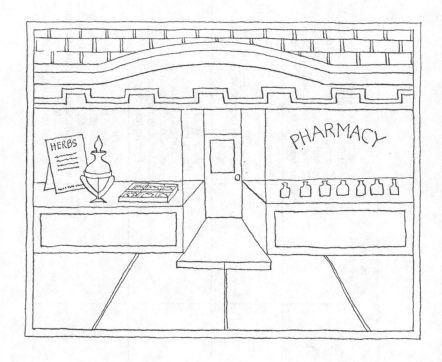

HERBS

If you can't grow and dry your own herbs, it is easy to get them ready dried. Some, like rosemary and sage, you can buy at the grocer's. Health food shops are proliferating all over the world, even in small towns, and if you ask in your local shop, you may find they sell herbs or know of a dried herb source near where you live. Otherwise, mail order sources often appear in health magazines; or you can try one of the following addresses:

SOURCES

Herbs

Wide World of Herbs Ltd.
11 St. Catherine Street East
Montreal 129, Canada
   This is one of the biggest dried herb sources available. The prices are quite competitive.

Indiana Botanic Gardens, Inc.
626 Seventeenth Street
Hammond, Indiana 46325
   The brochure and almanac issued by this company include descriptions of many herbs, oils, resins. Good fast-moving stock to choose from.

Herb Products Company, Inc.
11012 Magnolia Boulevard
North Hollywood, California 91601
   Excellent black and white drawings of many herbs from this wholesale-retail outlet. Aromatic mixtures and essential oils available too.

Nature's Herb Company
281 Ellis Street
San Francisco, California 94102

In addition to herbs the potpourris are available by ounce or pound. Essential oils.

Aphrodesia
28 Carmine Street
New York, New York 10014

A mixed bag of herbs and spices, some of which are appropriate to cosmetic and health care. Many descriptions of herbs. List of herbal books to purchase.

Harvest Health, Inc.
1944 Eastern Avenue S.E.
Grand Rapids, Michigan 49507

No brochure.

Kiehl's Pharmacy
109 Third Avenue
New York, New York 10003

An old-fashioned pharmacy with an excellent stock in herbs, oils, essences. No mail-order brochure, but you can write with specific rquests.

Wells Sweep Herb Farm
451 Mount Bethel Road
Port Murray, New Jersey 07865

No brochure.

Meadowbrook Herb Garden
Wyoming, Rhode Island 02898

Organically grown herbs, seeds, seaweed, teas and many herb books. Excellent brochure. This company packages well and is frequently distributed in health food stores.

Northwestern Processing Company
217 North Broadway
Milwaukee, Wisconsin 53202
    No brochure.

Lhasa Karnak Herb Company
2482 Telegraph Avenue
Berkeley, California 94704
    No brochure.

Rocky Hollow Herb Farm
Lake Walkill Road
Sussex, New Jersey 07461
    Organic supplies, dried flowers, roots, barks, berries, beans
and many cosmetic herbs, oils. Soapwort for shampoo, pine needle and oak bark for bath.

Oak Ridge Organic Herb Farm
P. O. Box 1055
Alton, Illinois 62002
    A wide variety of dried herbs and herb seeds, books, teas
and herbal advice, especially about comfrey.

Napier & Sons
17 Bristo Place
Edinburgh Ehl, Scotland
    Some unusual herbs and products and low prices. Send inter-
national reply coupon if you want an answer.

Potpourri Ingredients and Scents

Culpeper Limited
21 Bruton Steet
London W IX 8DS
England

Culpeper was the distinguished seventeenth-century herbalist, and the Society of Herbalists runs this and other Culpeper shops. Excellent toilet waters, creams and herbal preparations.

Caswell-Massey Co. Ltd.
Catalogue Order Department
320 West Thirteenth Street
New York, New York 10014

One of America's oldest apothecaries, on 518 Lexington Avenue, New York, has a unique and fascinating Victorian type catalogue of international and natural toiletries. Premixed potpourri or individual ingredients, perfume oils, soluble diluents, lavender water.

P. Fioretti & Company
1470 Lexington Avenue
New York, New York 10028

Company specializes in fragrances, essences and all materials for creating personal perfumes. Some prepared mixtures duplicate name-brand perfumes if you don't want to make your own.

Haussmann's Pharmacy
534 West Girard Avenue
Philadelphia, Pennsylvania 19123

One of the few mail order sources of Father Kneipp plant juices including nettle. Many of these juices are sleep, hair, skin aids. Cosmetic herbs, medicinal herbs and potpourri ingredients.

Caprilands Herb Farm
Silver Street
North Coventry, Connecticut 06238
Dried flowers for potpourri, hop pillow, fixatives and essential oils.

The Soap Box at Truc
40 Brattle Street
Cambridge, Massachusetts 12138
An interesting perfume burner, oils, soaps and natural toiletries.

Face and Body Shop
217 Newbury Street
Boston, Massachusetts 02116
A thoughtful collection of cosmetic herbs and oils and natural hair and body products. An indication of the national trend for special shops in this area.

Erewhon
Newbury Street
Boston, Massachusetts 02115. Also Los Angeles, California 90048
A remarkable country-store atmosphere in this large whole-sale-retail outlet. Some selection of dried herbs, large selection of natural products including a unique eggplant and salt tooth-powder. Herb books on the shelf.

Plants

Gardens of the Blue Ridge
Ashford, North Carolina 28603

Clyde Robin
P. O. Box 2091
Castro Valley, California 94546

Wild flowers are herbs—often herbs you can use for cosmetic and medicinal purposes. Highly recommended source for wild flower seed.

Theodore Payne Foundation
10459 Turford Street
Sun Valley, California 91352

California wild flowers and plants.

Nichols Garden Nursery
1190 North Pacific Highway
Albany, Oregon 97321

Besides selling peppermint oil straight from the peppermint fields of Oregon, Mr. Nichols sells a long list of hard-to-get herb plants. Shipping of herb plants starts April 1 and continues until June 15. Herbal books and gardening materials too.

Logee's Greenhouses
Danielson, Connecticut 06239

A large selection of herb plants.

The Tool Shed Herb Farm
Salem Center
Purdy's Station, New York 10578

A substantial selection of whole plants.

Merry Gardens
Camden, Maine 04843

Large mail order of herb plants and herb seeds.

Greene Herb Gardens
Greene, Rhode Island 02827
  Herb seeds.

Sparka's Woodland Acres Nursery
Crivitz, Wisconsin 54114
  Hardy wild flowers and fern with directions on planting.

Julius Roehrs Company
Rutherford, New Jersey, 07070
  Exotic plants.

Shirley Morgan
Mail Box Seeds
2042 Encinal Avenue
Alameda, California 94501
  Herb seeds. Send self-addressed envelope when making inquiries.

Vita-Green Farms, Inc.
P. O. Box 878
Vista, California 92083
  Mostly vegetable seeds, some herb seed. If you are into gardening, ecology, pure water you must write to Mr. Kinney and ask for his literature.

Growing Plants

House Plant Corner
P. O. Box 810
Oxford, Maryland 21654
  Supplies, materials for growing plants in the home under lights.

Hydroponics As a Hobby
University of Illinois
College of Agriculture
Extension Service in Agriculture and Home Economics
Urbana, Illinois 61801

This booklet will give you a start in this interesting science of growing things without soil.

Miscellaneous

Walnut Acres
Penns Creek, Pennsylvania 17862

Organic and natural foods from a long established, reputable house.

Lecithin:
American Lecithin Company
32-30 Sixty-first Street
Woodside, New York 11377

Purified Lanolin:
Kiehl's Pharmacy (see earlier listing)
Caswell-Massey (see earlier listing)

Wholesale:
Croda, Inc.
51 Madison Avenue, New York
New York, New York 10011

Rita Chemical Company
612 North Michigan Avenue
Chicago, Illinois 60611

CHAPTER XIII

BOTANICAL, PHARMACEUTICAL, FOOD USAGE CHART

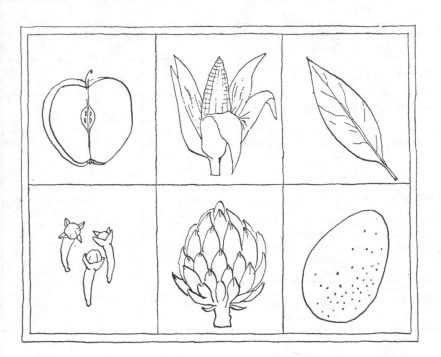

Herb	Skin	Hair	Eyes	Mouth	Feet
Almond meal	facial roughness, dryness, wrinkles, blackheads	-			
Almond oil	lotion	conditioner, growth			
Alum	tightener	darken hair			
Angelica					
Anise	.				
Apple	dryness, pimples			mouthwash	
Apricot	facial, vitamin A				
Artichoke		darken hair, growth			
Avocado	facial dryness, nourish-ment, cleanser	conditioner, shampoo			
Bay					
Balsam of Gilead	circulation, tightener, wrinkles, facial				
Barley	facial, wrinkles, pimples				
Bay leaf					
Bayberry 1) bark 2) root				X	
Bentonite	facial, thickener, healing				

Nails	Hands	Deodorant	Bath	Sleep	Astringent	Miscel-laneous
	lotion					scrub, external
	aid.					
				pillow		
				tablets		
				X		
						external
						external
	condi-tioner					external
						aroma
						external
						scrub, external
					X	
					X	

Herb	Skin	Hair	Eyes	Mouth	Feet
Benzoin	tightener, circulation, wrinkles, blemishes, cleanser				
Bindweed					swollen feet
Biotin		growth			
Birch sap	blemishes				
Bistort root				tooth powder	
Blackberry leaf					
Black cohosh					
Blackstrap molasses		growth, internal			
Borax	bleach, softener				
Boric acid powder			X		powder
Bouncing bet (soapwort)					
Boxwood shavings		X			
Bran	facial, large pores, dryness, tightening				
Brandy	oiliness, chap, roughness	oiliness			
Brewer's yeast	acne, pimples, eczema, oiliness, dryness, secretions of the skin, facial	problems		creases	

Nails	Hands	Deodorant	Bath	Sleep	Astringent	Miscellaneous
						aroma fixative, simple tincture
						internal
						internal
					X	
			X external			menstruation, internal
				X		internal
	cream		softener			external
						soap
		internal				cleanse, external
			scrub			external
	lotion					external
split nails, hangnails		internal				internal, external

Herb	Skin	Hair	Eyes	Mouth	Feet
Burdock root	acne				
Buttermilk	facial, bleaching, tightening, large pores, sunburn, oiliness				
Cactus					
Calamus root					
Calcium		external			
Camphor (gum)	facial, tightener, soothing, large pores	reviver		toothpaste	
Carbonate of soda					
Carnation					
Carrot	facial, pimples, vitamin A				
Cassia bud					
Castor oil	liver, age spots	strength-ener, con-ditioner, reviver			
Catechu		hair dye			
Catnip		dandruff, external			swelling, internal
Cat's tail	blemishes				swelling, internal
Cayenne pepper				gargle	powder for warmth
Celandine			X	X	

Nails	Hands	Deodorant	Bath	Sleep	Astringent	Miscellaneous
						cleanser, internal
						external
				internal		
						potpourri
aid internal				tablets, internal		
		internal				
			stimulating			external
						aroma
						internal, external
						aroma
						external

Herb	Skin	Hair	Eyes	Mouth	Feet
Celery	pimples		X		
Chamomile	facial, wrinkles, soothing, external	blond rinse, blond dye	compress, soothes puffiness		
Chickweed	freckles				
Chicory			strength- ener		
Chlorogalum	soap	shampoo			
Chrysan- themum					
Cinnamon					
Cleavers					
Clove		growth, external		mouthwash	
Cocoa butter	facial, creams, stretch marks	conditioner			
Coconut		shampoo			
Collard greens	internal				
Coltsfoot	veins				
Comfrey	facial, healing wrinkles, regenerates new cells		cream		
Cornmeal	cleanser, facial, large pores, soother, scrub				
Costmary					
Couch grass	blemish				swelling

Nails	Hands	Deodorant	Bath	Sleep	Astringent	Miscellaneous
						internal
			soothing, external	tea, internal	X	insect bites, external
			X			external
						internal
		X				
				X		potpourri
		X				
				internal		aroma
	lotion					
	healing					
			body cleanser			external
						aroma
						internal

Herb	Skin	Hair	Eyes	Mouth	Feet
Cowslip (English)	whitener, wrinkles				
Cramp bark					leg cramps
Cranberry juice	moles, external				
Cresses	salve, blemishes				
Cuckoopint	blemishes, cleanser				
Cucumber	cooling, tightening, nourishing, large pores, oiliness		soothing		
Daisy	pimples, blotches				
Damiana					
Dandelion	internal				
Dogwood twig				toothbrush, tooth whitener	
Egg white	facial, tightener, large pores, wrinkles, pimples, puffiness, sunburn, oiliness				
Egg yolk	facial, dry skin, conditioner	conditioner			
Elder 1) berry		black dye			X

Nails	Hands	Deodorant	Bath	Sleep	Astringent	Miscel-laneous
						cleanser
						internal
				internal		
					pore tightener	external
				X		
					pore tightener	external
	X					external

Herb	Skin	Hair	Eyes	Mouth	Feet
Elder 2) flower	facial, complexion waters, bleach, wrinkles, blemishes		healer		
3) leaf					powder
Endive			internal		
Epsom salt	double chin bandage, blackheads				
Escarole			strengthener		
Eucalyptus					
Eyebright			wash, inflammation, puffiness		
Fennel	facial wrinkles, impurities		compress		
Fern					foot bath, cures fatigue, leg cramps
Fig			X		
Flaxseed (linseed)	softener in facial	setting lotion	compress		
Folic acid		internal			
Fuller's earth	thickener for facial	dry shampoo			
Garlic					corn

Nails	Hands	Deodorant	Bath	Sleep	Astringent	Miscellaneous
			curative, stimulating, soothing	X		external
			curative, relieves aches			external
						internal
			curative, body aches			
						internal, external
			curative			external
						constipation
barrier, protective cream						

Herb	Skin	Hair	Eyes	Mouth	Feet
Gelatine	thickener for facial	setting lotion, gives body			.
Geranium					swelling
Gladwin	sores, itches, scabs				
Glycerine	facial, moisturizing emollient, double chin bandage, healing			.	
Goldenrod					
Goldensea	healer		compress		X
Grape	dry skin, tan, sunburn, freckles, external				
Grapefruit					
Gum arabic	tightener	setting lotion			
Gum tragacanth	facial tightener, large pores			X	
Hay flower	curative				problems
Heliotrope					
Henna		hair dye			
Holm oak		darken hair			
Honey	facial, healing, moisturizing, wrinkles, blackheads, large pores, nourishing, external	blond dye		.	

Nails	Hands	Deodorant	Bath	Sleep	Astringent	Miscellaneous
internal strengthener						
						external
	lotion, healing					
			external			
				internal		
				hot juice		
					X	aroma fixative
					X	aroma fixative, scent balls
			curative			
						aroma
nail dye						
nail aid			nourishing	retains body fluids, internal		with apple cider is reviving, internal

Herb	Skin	Hair	Eyes	Mouth	Feet
Hops					
Horse-radish	bleaching (grated), acne (compound spirit)				
Horsetail	facial, large pores, oiliness, internal, external		reduces swelling, external		stimulating, external
Houseleek	facial, wrinkles, healing, nourishing creams				corn
Indian corn	blemishes				swelling
Inositol		anti-grey, aids growth			
Irish moss	softener for facial	setting lotion			
Ivy twig	sunburn				
Jaborandi		growth stimulating			
Jasmine					
Juniper					
Kaolin	thickener in facial	filler for dye			
Karaya Gum	tightener	setting lotion			
Kelp		oiliness			

Nails	Hands	Deodorant	Bath	Sleep	Astringent	Miscellaneous
				tea in pillows		
						external
regenerates, external			curative, stimulating, external		X	
						external
						internal
			X			aroma
				X		
	protective in cream					
					X	
						use instead of salt

Herb	Skin	Hair	Eyes	Mouth	Feet
Lady's mantle (whole herb)	facial, lotion, creams, acne, wrinkles, inflammation				
Lady's slipper					
Lamb's quarters (pigweed)	cleanser				
Lanolin	facial, creams, moisturizer, emollient, wrinkles				
Laurel		darkens hair			
Lavender water/oil		wash		clean teeth, gargle	cures fatigue
Lecithin	facial, acne				
Lemon	facial, spring cleaner, restores acidity, large pores, oiliness, blackheads, external	setting lotion, external		tooth cleaner, external	
Lemon balm					
Lemon verbena					

Nails	Hands	Deodorant	Bath	Sleep	Astringent	Miscellaneous
	X		soothing	tea under pillow promotes sleep	very astringent	can flush kidneys, external, internal
				X		
						soap
			liquid			
		external	aroma	pillow		aroma, headache, depression tonic, fever, external
cuticle aid, external				hot lemonade, internal		
				tea, internal; pillows, external		
				tea, internal; pillow, external		

Herb	Skin	Hair	Eyes	Mouth	Feet
Lettuce, cultivated	eau de laitre, complexion water				
Lettuce, wild					
Lilac flower	cleans, softens				
Lily of the valley					
Lime flower (linden)	facial, wrinkles, large pores, plant hormones, impurities, external				
Linseed (see Flaxseed)					
Liver	pimples	X			
Logwood		darkens hair			
Lovage					
Lupine seed	blemishes, external				
Magnesium		needed			
Maidenhair fern		growth			
Marigold (calendula)	facial, thread veins, healing, wrinkles	red dye	lotion		
Marjoram					
Marshmallow 1) flower 2) root	facial lotion, roughness	hair lightener lotion			

Nails	Hands	Deodorant	Bath	Sleep	Astringent	Miscellaneous
		internal, external		tea		
				tea		
						use as soap
						aroma
			curative	tea		cleanses system, tranquilizes, internal
						internal
		external				
						internal
						aroma

Herb	Skin	Hair	Eyes	Mouth	Feet
Melon	dry skin				
Milk	facial, healing, dry skin, rough skin, acne, oiliness, external				
Mint	facial, stimulating, cleansing, external			mouthwash, external	
Mulberry		darken hair			
Mullein		lighten hair			
Mushroom					
Musk					
Myrrh	facial, healing, wrinkles			stimulating to membranes, mouthwash	
Myrtle	blemishes	darken hair			
Narcissus root	facial				
Nettle	facial, cleanser, stimulating, soothing, impurities, plant hormones, external	reviver, dandruff, growth, external	X external	breath sweetener, internal	
Nutmeg		growth		mouthwash	
Oak bark	X				
Oak moss					

Nails	Hands	Deodorant	Bath	Sleep	Astringent	Miscellaneous
			soothing, external	with honey, internal		
			soothing, healing, external			aroma, soothing, cleansing, internal, tea
		internal				
			X			aroma fixative
					X	
						potpourri
	chap chaser					potpourri
		internal	curative		X	
				X		aroma
						scent powder

Herb	Skin	Hair	Eyes	Mouth	Feet
Oat flower	impurities				foot bath problems
Oatmeal	facial, soothing, whitening, blackheads, healing, external				
Olive oil	nourishing, sunburn	nourishing, conditioner			
Onion	blemishes, spots, wrinkles				corn
Orange flower					
Orrisroot		dry shampoo			
PABA	sunburn ointment, external	restorer, growth, internal			
Pantothenic acid		growth, internal			
Papaya	facial, dead skin cleanser external		dark circles, external		
Parsley	facial, thread veins, external	sheen, conditioner, external	compress	breath sweetener, internal	
Parsnip		hair conditioner			
Passion flower					
Patchouli oil					
Patience	pimples				

Nails	Hands	Deodorant	Bath	Sleep	Astringent	Miscellaneous
			curative			
	lotion		soothing, healing, relieves itching			non-aller-genic scrub or soap
conditioner						
						external
				tea, internal		aroma
				pillow		fixative, potpourri
		internal				
				X		
		external				aroma

Herb	Skin	Hair	Eyes	Mouth	Feet
Peach 1) fruit 2) leaf	facial moisturizer	reviver, shampoo			
Pellitory of the wall	spots, freckles, pimples, sunburn				
Pennyroyal					
Peppermint	facial, stimulating, tightening, external				
Pimpernel	blemishes, complexion water				
Pineapple juice					
Pine needles					
Plantain (common)	healing		compress		
Plum	X				
Potato	facial, cleansing, nourishing, maintaining, bleach, oiliness, sunburn, external; eczema, internal		puffiness		
Privit		golden dye with radish			
Pulsatilla					

Nails	Hands	Deodorant	Bath	Sleep	Astringent	Miscellaneous
				tea		
				tea, internal; pillow, external		aroma, internal cleanser, calming, soothing
			X			
X						
			eases body aches			
			X			can stop bleeding
				X		

Herb	Skin	Hair	Eyes	Mouth	Feet
Quassia chips		rinse for dark hair, sheen			
Quebracho		darken hair			
Quince seed	softener for facial	growth, setting lotion, golden hair dye			
Radish		golden hair dye			
Raspberry	cleansing, internal			compress	
Red bergamot					
Red Clover	skin eruptions				
Red robin (geranium)					reduces swelling, external
Redwood		darken hair			
Restharrow					internal
Rhubarb root		golden hair dye			
Riboflavin	brown spots, internal				
Rose 1) water 2) bud	creams, facial bleaching			mouthwash	
Rose geranium					
Rose hip tea	bleaching freckles		puffiness, dark circles		

Nails	Hands	Deodorant	Bath	Sleep	Astringent	Miscellaneous
		tops				
			nourisher			menstrual problems, childbirth
				tea		
			X			
lotion			X			
				in pillows		aroma
						aroma
						internal

Herb	Skin	Hair	Eyes	Mouth	Feet
Rosemary	facial	dandruff, hair wash, setting lotion, reviver, lustre, curls			
Rue (flower)	pimples				
Rum		oily hair, external			
Safflower oil	facial				
Saffron		reddish-blond dye			
Sage	large pores, facial, external	dandruff, darken hair wash		tooth whitener, mouthwash, cleaner	
Salt	invigorating			mouthwash, tooth cleaner	
Sassafras bark	acne		X		
Sesame oil	lotion, suntan facial				
Silver mantle	blemishes				swelling
Silverweed	blemishes, sunburn, pimples, freckles				
Skullcap					
Soapberry					
Southernwood		shampoo, rinse for dark hair			
Soybean		oiliness, internal			

Nails	Hands	Deodorant	Bath	Sleep	Astringent	Miscellaneous
			cleanser, eases body aches	pillows		
				X		
			X			
		controls perspiration	curative	tea, internal; pillow, external		
			before bath body rub			
			X			
						impurities
				tea, internal		
						soap

Herb	Skin	Hair	Eyes	Mouth	Feet
Spike					
Storax					
Strawberry	clears oiliness, internal, external		X	tooth cleaner	
Sulphur water	liver, brown spots, acne, pimples, external				
Sunflower seed and oil	cleanser, nourisher, high in lecithin			strengthens teeth	
Sweet cream	facial, wrinkles, nourishing, external				
Swiss Kriss		darkens hair			
Tag alder root		darkens hair			
Tarragon					
Teasel			X		
Thyme	facial				
Tomato	facial, large pores, nourishing				
Tonquin					
Turkey oil					

Nails	Hands	Deodorant	Bath	Sleep	Astringent	Miscellaneous
						aroma
						aroma fixative
			X		lotion	
						high in vitamin A, E, calcium, phosphorus, fluorine
						herbal laxative product
				pillow		
						aroma
					X	
						aroma
			disperses in water			is treated castor oil

Herb	Skin	Hair	Eyes	Mouth	Feet
Turnip top				breath sweetener, internal	
Valerian					
Vervain					
Vetiver					
Vinegar	cleanser, softener, itchiness, flakiness, sunburn, large pores, blackheads, anti-fatigue	dandruff, conditioner, rinse			itchiness
Violet water			compress		
Vitamin A	rough skin, acne, blemishes, infection			gum aid	
Vitamin B complex	dermatitis, dry, scaly	needed		aids receding gums	
Vitamin B_2	liver spots				
Vitamin B_{12}	eczema				
Vitamin C	infection, black and blue marks			swollen gums, pulp of teeth	leg cramps
Vitamin D					

Nails	Hands	Deodorant	Bath	Sleep	Astringent	Miscellaneous
		internal				.
				capsule or tea		
				internal		
		suppresses perspiration				
strengthens			invigorating, lessens fatigue			apple cider preferred
growth						
strengthens		foods containing B are antiperspirant				
ridges						

Herb	Skin	Hair	Eyes	Mouth	Feet
Vitamin E	facial, moisturizer, wrinkles, chin aid, brown liver spots, circulation, internal, external, burns, heals wounds				
Walnut shell		dyes hair darker			
Watercress	blemishes, internal, external				
Wheat germ	facial, thread veins, allergic skin, internal, external				
Wheat germ oil	nourishing, dry skin, chin and neck, allergic skin				
Wild pansy	blemishes				
Willow 1) bark 2) leaves 3) sap	spots dis-colouring	dandruff			bath for weak feet
Wine (white)	blackheads, oiliness, external	wash external			

Nails	Hands	Deodorant	Bath	Sleep	Astringent	Miscel-laneous
						blood cleanser
			recovering illness			

Herb	Skin	Hair	Eyes	Mouth	Feet
Witch hazel	sunburn, puffiness, tightener		puffiness, inflammation, dark circles		
Wood moss					foot bath, leg cramps, fallen arches
Woodruff					
Wormwood	healing, eruptions, scabs, eczema				
Yarrow	facial, dilates pores, cuts grease, internal, external	oiliness			
Yogurt	facial, normal-oily, cleanser, bleach, external				
Yucca	soap	shampoo			

Nails	Hands	Deodorant	Bath	Sleep	Astringent	Miscel-laneous
					pore tightener	
				tea, internal; pillow, external		
					cuts grease	heals wounds, sore nipples

INDEX

aches, *see* eucalyptus; pine needles

acne, 41, 42; causes, 43; *see also* lady's mantle

adolescence, 41–42

alder root, to darken hair, 119

almond meal, in bath, 89; for large pores, 54; skin cleanser, 17; scrub, 51

almond oil, for blackheads, 44; hair conditioner, 97; for hair growth, 111; for hands, 134, 136; skin nourisher, 56, 58, 61–65

ambergris, in bath, 85; in scent, 162

alum, to darken hair, 119; skin tightener, 54, 56

angelica pillow, 153

anise, for sleep, 152

aniseed, for sleep, 152

antibiotics, *see* drugs

apple, mouthwash, 130; for dry skin, 58; for rough skin, 61; for sleep, 153

arches, fallen, 144–45

artichokes, to darken hair, 118; for hair growth, 110, 112

astringents, 72–75

attar of roses, 162

avocado oil, in bath, 87; hair conditioner, 97; for nails, 139; shampoo, 96; skin (cleanser) 16, (dry skin) 58, (nourisher) 24

bacteria, 7, 94; *see also* toxins

balm, to darken hair, 119

balsam of Gilead, skin tightener, 12

baths, basic needs, 83; for circulation, 82, 91; cold, 92; for energy, 82; expensive, 90; friction, 91; nourishing, 87; for relaxation, 82; salt toner, 91; for sleep, 149–50; soothing and toning, 89–92; *see also* feet

bayberry bark, astringent, 75

bayberry root, for teeth, 129

bay essence, in bath, 85

bay leaves, in potpourri, 161

bay salt, in potpourri, 160

bean shells, to darken hair, 119

bee balm, in potpourri, 161; tea, for sleep, 152

beets, as deodorants, 79; for breath, 131

benzoin, astringent, 12; for circulation, 34; for double chin, 68; in potpourri, 160; in scent, 163

betony, to darken hair, 119

bicarbonate of soda, in bath, 90

bindweed, for swollen feet, 145

birch, for skin blemishes, 48

bistort root, astringent, 75; for teeth, 129

blackberry leaves, in bath, 90

blackheads, 43–49

blemishes, 11; causes, 82, 41–42; control, 43–49; *see also* acne; spots

body temperature, 7, 83

borax, skin softener, 23

boric acid, for eyes, 123

boxwood shavings, for hair growth, 110

bran, in bath, 89; face scrub, 51; for large pores, 54; skin cleanser, 15

brandy, for chapped skin, 61; for hands, 133–34

brazil wood, hair dye, 115

breath, 131; *see also* parsley

brewer's yeast, for acne, 42; deodorant, 78; for double chin, 67; for grey hair, 113; for hair, 94–95; for nails, 138; for skin, 50, 53, 58, 64; for thread veins, 64; for wrinkles, 21

brown spots, 50

buckbush, in soap, 20

burns, *see* comfrey

buttermilk, for large pores, 54, 55; skin bleach, 49, 53, 70; oily skin, 52

cabbage, for oily skin, 52

calamus root, in potpourri, 161

ACKNOWLEDGEMENTS

For invaluable help in research and preparation for this book I have to thank Alexander Dubenchiek, who kept me informed on the chemistry of the herbs. Ira Kapp, president of Felton International generously supplied me with most of the oils, perfumes and materials for making lotions and creams. Vivienne Heisler shared her time, wit and intelligence. The book is far better for her interest and efforts.

Elizabeth Hall, senior librarian of the Horticultural Society of New York; Julia Weiss of the Mahopac Library and Mid-Hudson System; the librarians of the New York Academy of Medicine; Dorothy Gomez of the Royal Horticultural Society of London; and Phoebe Abelow; Shirley and Milton Asnis; Marilyn and David Balk; Harriet Berchenko; Frank Berchenko, M.D.; Sonny Caldwell; Mary Campbell; Diane Cleaver; Sidney Darion; Stephanie Delan; Anita Diamant; Emma Fisher; Anna and Colin Haycraft; Judith Kardish; Helen and Boris Kaufman; Beth Merritt; Susan Meyer; Jonathan Miller; Antoine Millet; Jean Mundy; Susan Neumann and Dossie Tannor were all helpful in the research and preparation.

Finally my deepest debt is due to members of my family: my grandmother Anna-Pearl, whose knowledge of herbal lore, particularly gypsy herbal secrets, started me in my own lifelong pursuit; and her daughter, my mother, Renee Dincin, to whom this book is dedicated; Edward Dincin; Zola Dincin Schneider; Daniel Schneider; Norman Schneider; my husband, Herman Buchman, whose support has been constant and unfailing, and whose practical knowledge of the human face, derived from his work as a stage and film make-up man, has been most useful; and my daughter Cathleen, who is an enthusiastic herbalist and fellow experimenter.